BACK CHAT BEAUTY

First published in the United Kingdom in 2019 by
Pavilion
43 Great Ormond Street
London
WC1N 3HZ

The publishers would like to thank Shutterstock®, Adam Hale and Peter Pedonomou for their kind permission to reproduce the illustrations in this book. Every effort has been made to trace the copyright holders and obtain permission to reproduce this material. However, the publishers will be glad to rectify in future editions any inadvertent omissions brought to their attention.

ISBN 978-1-91162-464-6

A CIP catalogue record for this book is available from the British Library.

10 9 8 7 6 5 4 3 2 1

Reproduction by Rival Colour Ltd, UK
Printed and bound by Toppan Leefung Printing Ltd, China

www.pavilionbooks.com

BACK CHAT BEAUTY

The Beauty Guide for Real Life

Sophie Beresiner and
Lisa Potter-Dixon

PAVILION

THE BACK

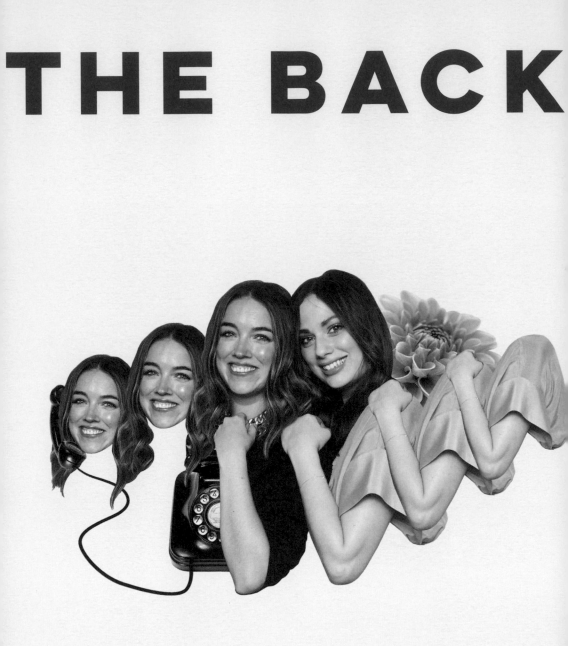

CHAT

Backchat Beauty started as just that, a chat. This chat in fact:

> *L.P.D.* Soph, get out of your pyjamas. I'm gonna add you to my Instagram LIVE in a minute. Collectively we've got 30 years of beauty experience between us – that is a LOT. Might as well share it. You do the beauty editor point of view, I'll do the makeup artist point of view, and we can just chat beauty.

> *S.B.* Erm... YES! Argh! I'd better put my face on.

> No! Do it LIVE! This'll be real.

↳ Hi guys, get ready with me live with @sophieberesiner

1 HOUR LATER

> That was amazing! We should make it a regular thing – maybe one day it could be a book, imagine! Laterz, I'm going to spin.

1 WEEK LATER

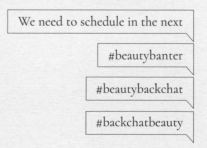

> We need to schedule in the next

> #beautybanter

> #beautybackchat

> #backchatbeauty

Yes we do! Oooooooooh FAVE so far...

#backchatbeauty

Sold! OK, have to go, I'm having copper leaf applied on my nails so I can't type.

1 YEAR LATER

Soph, got the deadline for the book! Let's make it the most honest and useful beauty book we can possibly imagine.

Exciting! Has to be a comprehensive guide that covers everything from the basics, so people can nail their base, brows, eyes, lips, hair, the works, but then we should cover the sh*t people don't talk about. The stuff that messes with your makeup, like crying... or rain. Or childbirth!

IMHO

And hangovers and heartbreak. What is IMHO?

I've definitely got some funny stories I can add in and I know you have too, like what happened when you first wore red lipstick. I love that one.

In My Humble Opinion. Really Lise...

It'll be real advice from real women for real women. Done! We can ask our expert friends for their ultimate tips. And travel – we've got to do an Out-Of-Office section.

Don't forget The Good Times. We can talk about weddings, work, love, going out, staying in – PLEASE put your baked Camembert recipe in there somewhere.

It's a lot to fit in one book. We're going to need prosecco. And coffee.

ANOTHER YEAR LATER

Fifty-eight thousand coffees, several gallons of prosecco, a weekend in Margate and a lot of laughing helped us get our very best combined advice down on these pages.

Starting with the basics, you'll be able to pick the right products to nail your base, map your brows and even master the best eye looks (IMHO). We'll also help you win at REAL LIFE. Real life isn't what you see in magazines, on TV or even on Instagram. Real life is about the good times, the good-time disruptors and getting it right in and out of the office! We've shared our own stories from our real lives to create what we think is genuinely the most useful book we could, and we hope you agree.

So whether you're in love, looking for love, caught in the rain or heading to the beach, you'll find everything you ever wanted to know about looking GREAT in these pages. Remember, it's only makeup (but we bloody love it). Over to you... #backchatbeauty.

THE BASI

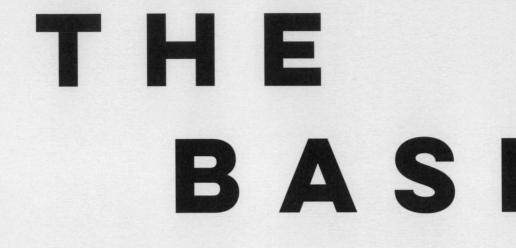

THIS IS THE ESSENTIAL STUFF –
NECESSARY AND USEFUL GO-TO
TIPS THAT COVER EVERYTHING
FROM YOUR EYEBROWS DOWN.
IT'S SIMPLIFIED BUT COMPREHENSIVE.
WE'VE GOT YOU.

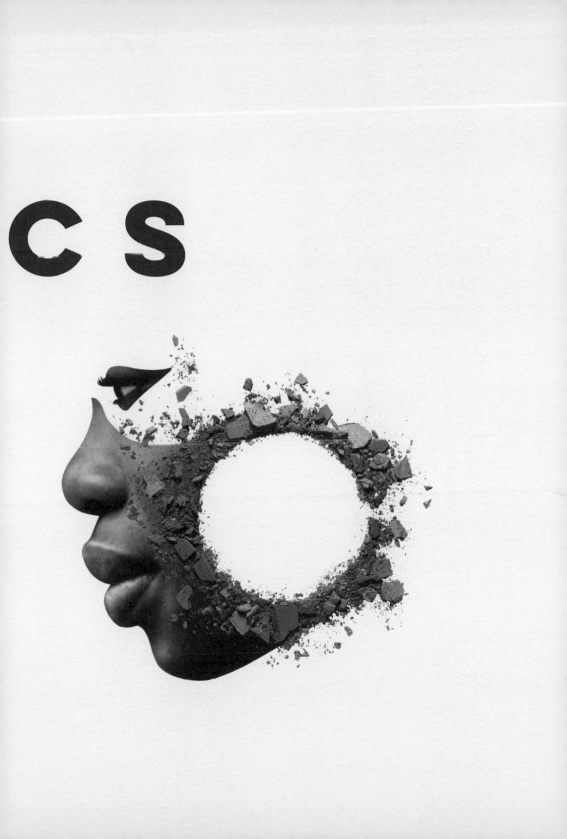

YOUR BASE

IMPORTANT BECAUSE

IT'S THE ONE THING THAT CAN MAKE
YOU LOOK WAY OLDER OR WAY YOUNGER
THAN YOU ARE DEPENDING ON HOW IT'S APPLIED.

IT HAS THE POWER TO HIDE
OR HIGHLIGHT SKIN DILEMMAS OR SINS.

AN EVEN COMPLEXION IS A
SIGNIFIER FOR GOOD HEALTH.

PICK YOUR FINISH

MATTE

These products will leave you free from shine and offer a bit more coverage.

Good for:
• Oily skin.
• Excess shine.
• Full coverage.
• Longwear.

Not so good for:
• Dry skin.
• Older skin.
• A natural look.

SHEER

You can see your skin through these products, so if you've got a great complexion, flaunt it!

Good for:
• No-makeup makeup.
• Sundays.
• Hot weather and holidays.
• Freckles.

Not so good for:
• Problem skin.
• Nights out.
• Oily skin.

DEWY

This is the 'lit from within' look.

Good for:
• Most people (it's Lisa's absolute fave).
• A healthy look.
• Natural glow.

Not so good for:
• Uneven-textured skin.

MINERAL

These products look natural and have serious skin health benefits.

Good for:
• Sophie (she is obsessed).
• Letting your skin breathe.
• Easy application.
• Sensitive skin.

Not so good for:
- Full coverage.
- Older skin (powder only).

> *L.P.D.* One of the biggest mistakes women make is to use a heavy foundation to cover a beauty dilemma, when in fact you should use a lighter foundation and let your concealer work its magic on your problem areas. If you absolutely have to use a base for confidence, try sheer base products or tinted moisturizer.

PERFECT YOUR BASE

HOW TO COVER SPOTS AND BLEMISHES

If you don't have to, don't wear makeup when you've got spots. Obviously that's not ideal, as you'll want to hide them to get on with real life. So when you do have to cover up, try pinpointing.

Pinpointing 101
- Use a clean fine eyeliner brush, dip it into a cream concealer, then dab it directly onto the spot.
- Use either a clean eyeshadow brush or clean fingers to pat the product into the skin until the spot disappears.
- Repeat if necessary.
- Wash your brushes well and leave to dry. Wash your hands well before you continue applying makeup.

HOW TO COVER UNDER THE EYE

There is no such thing as a creaseless concealer, particularly if you laugh a lot, but there are ways to ensure your concealer stays crease-free for longer. Like the V technique, below. Always use a concealer that is one shade lighter than your complexion to brighten around the eyes. But PLEASE do not use a highlighting concealer, which will only illuminate dark circles.

Some people have dark lids, too – feel free to conceal right from the lash line to your brow, which creates a great base for eye makeup and will really showcase the pigment in anything you use next.

The V technique
1. Using a liquid concealer and starting in the inner corner of your eye, draw a V shape under the eye, down to the apple of your cheek, then back to the outer corner of the eye.
2. Blend the product upwards toward the lower lash line – a damp Beautyblender is great for this. As are your fingers.

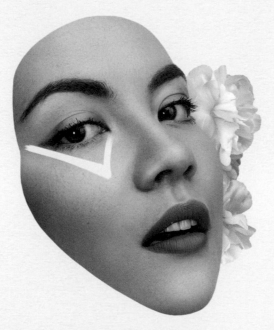

HOW TO COVER DISCOLOURATION

First things first: your face is not one colour. It's more like an impressionist painting if you really break it down. Also, it can change from day to day for various reasons. Like, for instance, stress, excitement, drinking alcohol, hormones, rosacea, sun damage, falling asleep on a newspaper (Sophie has done this). There are a few simple pigmented products here to help.

CONCEALING WITH COLOUR

Red	Cancels dark circles on deep skin tones.
Yellow	Calms mild redness on all skin tones.
Pink	Cancels dark circles and brightens dullness on fair skin tones.
Green	Calms the look of intense red areas on all skin tones.
Lilac	Cancels dark circles and brightens dullness on medium skin tones.
Orange	Cancels dark circles and combats dark spots on dark to deep skin tones.
Peach	Cancels dark circles and combats dark spots on light to medium skin tones.

Lisa's colour-correcting sandwich

1. Apply a base layer: the colour corrector (pick whichever product you need using the advice on page 17). This should go underneath your foundation because the colours are weird, and you don't want to see them once you've finished. Putting it directly on the dilemma means you'll make the most of the product.

2. Apply a middle layer: foundation. Use this to blend out the colour corrector, even-out and brighten (or mattify) your skin. Whatever your base, it shouldn't be the thing that 'conceals' the problem.

3. Apply a top layer: concealer. Finish by dotting concealer over any areas that need a little extra help, blending to perfection with a fluffy eyeshadow brush or damp Beautyblender.

YOUR
BROWS

IMPORTANT BECAUSE

YOUR BROWS FRAME AND BALANCE YOUR FACE.

THEY CAN OPEN YOUR EYES
AND MAKE YOU LOOK MORE AWAKE.

THEY CAN TAKE YEARS OFF
YOUR AGE, HONESTLY!

PICK YOUR PRODUCT

Powder	For a soft, natural finish.
Pencil	For definition and to fill any gaps.
Felt pen	For hair-like strokes.
Brow gel	Shape and set all in one.
Cream gel	For the Insta-brow.
Fibre gel	To add volume.

HOW TO MAP YOUR BROWS

Your brows should always start, arch and end in the right place. If they start in the right place then your nose will look slimmer. If they arch in the right place then your eyes will look more open. And if they end in the right place then your cheekbones will look lifted.

1. Hold a thin makeup brush or pencil at the corner of your nose and point it straight up to the ceiling. Where it hits your brow bone is where your brows should start. Make a small mark here with a brow pencil.

2. Keep the makeup brush or pencil at the corner of the nose, but this time, look straight ahead and angle it through the centre of your pupil. Where it hits your brow bone is where the brow should arch. Make another small mark.

3. Finally, angle the brush from the corner of your nose to the outer corner of your eye. Where it hits the brow bone is the perfect ending. Make a small mark and fill in your brows following the marks as a guide to the best possible shape.

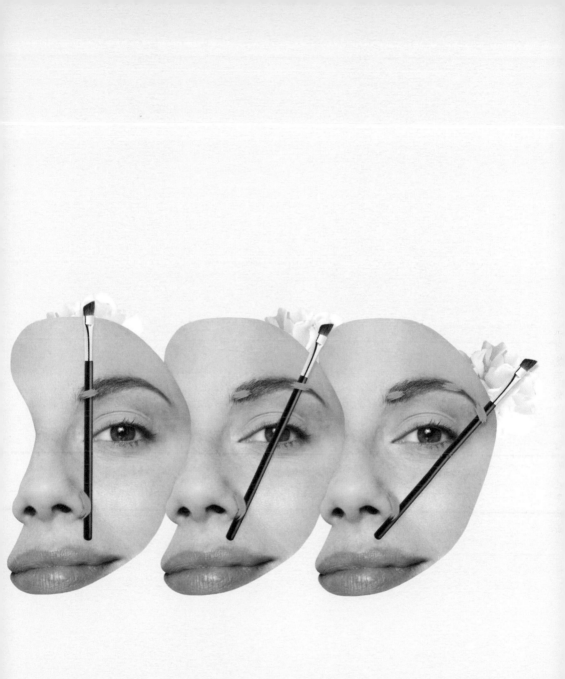

YOUR EYES

IMPORTANT BECAUSE

PEOPLE LOOK INTO THEM/GET LOST
IN THEM/AVOID THEM (DELETE AS APPROPRIATE)

BUT REALLY, IT'S THE PLACE PEOPLE LOOK
WHEN THEY TALK TO YOU SO MAKE THE MOST
OF THEM.

YOU CAN MAKE THEM APPEAR BIGGER,
SMALLER; MAKE YOURSELF SEEM MORE AWAKE –
IT'S GREAT FUN TO PLAY WITH!

MASCARA

DO ...

• Test a variety of mascaras to find the best product for you. Your friend's fave may not look the same on your lashes.
• Apply mascara to bottom lashes first, because you naturally look up when you do so, and if you've done the top, the mascara will transfer to your lids.
• Concentrate the product in the middle of your eyes to make them appear rounder, or concentrate it in the outer corner to make your lashes appear elongated.
• Try coloured mascara – it's an easy and often-overlooked way to change up your look.

DON'T ...

• Think one mascara size fits all – pick the right product using our tips below.
• Keep mascara for any longer than three months once opened. Bacterial infection warning!
• Rub mascara off – soak a cotton pad in eye makeup remover, hold on the lashes with your eyes closed for 30 seconds to dissolve the mascara, then wipe off gently.

MASCARA BY TYPE

Long, straight lashes	Try a curling mascara like Benefit Roller Lash, or curl your lashes before you apply any product.
Short, fine lashes	Try lengthening mascara like Clinique Lash Power Mascara and turn the wand vertically and use the tip to add length.

Curly lashes	Try volumizing mascara like Benefit BADgal BANG! to make the most of your natural lift.
Thick lashes	Try a lightweight, separating mascara like Glossier Lash Slick, otherwise they can clog together.
For all lashes	Try a tubing mascara like Pixi Beauty LashLift 188.

EYELINER

Difficulty rating:
* easy
** a little tricky
*** a bit harder

KOHL PENCIL (*)

This is best for a soft, smoky finish. Use it in the waterline to define your eyes, then add a line along the upper lash line. How much you use is up to you: a little at the corners can lift eyes, a full line can add definition and you can smudge it up with a cotton bud for a smouldering, easy-to-manage look.

GEL (***)

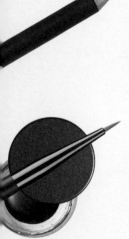

This is best for a defined, highly pigmented line. It will last the longest once applied so it's great for a night out! If you're thinking of trying a classic flick, this is the one you need. Gel liner can take a bit of practice to get right, so if you're trying it for the first time, then have a few practices without any other makeup first. This way you can wipe it away without having to start again.

LIQUID (**)

This is best for a fluid, solid line and can be used to create a classic flick if you're not confident with gel liner. Take it out with you for topping up throughout the day or night.

FELT-TIP (*)

This is best for a precise line of varying thickness and is GREAT for using on the move because you can apply it one-handed.

EYESHADOW

CREAM

Pros: Cream eyeshadow blends really easily, gives a dewy finish, is great for drier skin types and can be applied with fingers.
Cons: It is not as long-lasting as powder eyeshadow, it's less buildable and it creases easily, meaning you'll have to keep an eye on it.

POWDER

Pros: Powder eyeshadow comes in multiple textures – from matte to metallic, it's great for layering and blending, and good for oily eyelids, as it absorbs natural oils.
Cons: Watch out for 'fallout' under eyes with powder eyeshadow! It can feel dry or cause dryness and needs brushes for application.

THE LOOKS

HOW TO DO A CLASSIC SMOKE

You'll need two colours of eyeshadow, a kohl liner and a mascara.
1. Take the lighter colour and dust it all over your lid up to the socket. Keep your eye open to feel where your socket is.
2. Draw your kohl pencil along the lash line, get as close as you can but don't worry about being too precise. Buff this to give a smoky liner effect.
3. Take your darker shadow and buff from the outer corner of the eye, inwards, to about a third of the way in.
4. Blend a small amount of the darker shadow under the lower lash line. If you add too much, use the lighter shade over the top.
5. Finish by lining the waterline with the kohl pencil and then add loads of mascara.

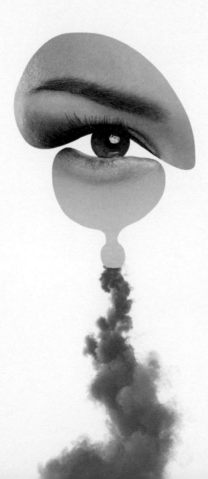

HOW TO DO A WINGED SMOKE

You'll need one eyeshadow colour for this look.

1. Using a fine eyeliner brush, draw outwards from the corner of your eye towards your brow, then return the line towards the outer third of your lash line in the shape of a V.

2. Fill in the V and blend very softly with a cotton bud for a soft winged smoke.

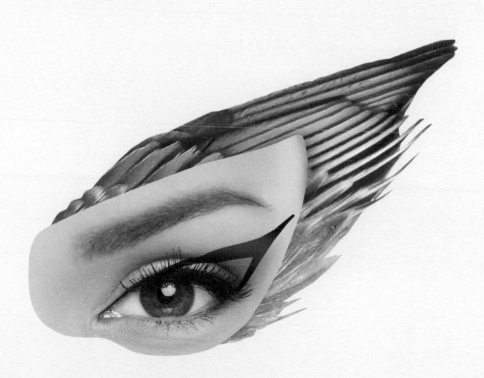

HOW TO DO A 'NO-SMOKE'

You can create this look using eyeshadow, lipstick, bronzer, whatever you have to hand.

1. Draw a 'C' shape, starting in the socket of your eyelid about halfway across the eye and down to the lash line.

2. Use a fluffy eyeshadow brush to blend the colour into the socket and along the lash line. Instant natural smoky eye!

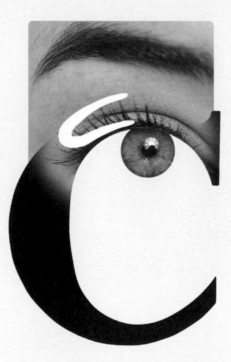

HOW TO DO SOPHIE'S LOOK: THE COOL CONTOUR

> *S.B.* If it's not easy, I'm not doing it.

1. Take a crayon eyeshadow and draw on a No-smoke (see opposite).
2. Blend the product into the eye using a fluffy eyeshadow brush and take it down beneath the lower lash line.
3. Add grey liquid liner to the upper lash line.
4. Douse lashes in mascara.

SOPHIE LOVES: Laura Mercier Caviar Stick Eye Colour in Taupe.

HOW TO DO LISA'S LOOK: THE DISCO BALL

> *L.P.D.* If in doubt, chuck on some glitter.

1. Apply bronzer from the lash line to the socket.
2. Dab full-on liquid glitter in the centre of the eyelid.
3. Add more and more until you feel like Cher!

LISA LOVES: Stila Magnificent Metals Glitter & Glow Liquid Eye Shadow in Rose Gold Retro.

YOUR CHEEKS

IMPORTANT BECAUSE

YOUR CHEEKS ARE BASICALLY RESPONSIBLE FOR HOW HEALTHY YOU DO OR DON'T LOOK.

COLOUR CAN RESTRUCTURE YOUR WHOLE FACE.

YOUR CHEEKS ARE THE HEART AND SOUL OF YOUR GLOWABILITY.

BLUSHER

Selecting a blush product is all about personal preference. But in general...

POWDER

Easy to build and blend, and probably the most popular option due to the variety of colours.

CREAM

Perfect for a dewy sheen of colour, easy to apply with fingers and great for a natural no-makeup makeup look.

STAIN

To create the perfect flush as if you've been out on a cold day.

WE LOVE: Benefit Benetint is the original cheek stain (est 1976) and still the best. It's easy to blend with fingers, a brush or sponge.

BRONZER

You should be wearing bronzer. Here's how.

MATTE

Good for using all over your face for a healthy glow, or to create shadow beneath cheekbones and in eye sockets.

SHIMMER

Use to accentuate your cheekbones and add some general fabulousness – also great on the eyelids.

STICK/CREAM

Great for a full-on contour as it blends beautifully, and can be used for more precise application – get drawing!

HIGHLIGHTER

You want glow, therefore you want highlighter.

CREAM

Great for a subtle glow as it's easy to blend.

POWDER

Buildable and excellent if you want your highlighter to be seen from space – it gives a 'dry-gloss' effect.

LIQUID

The most versatile highlighting product – a little goes a long way. Use it under your foundation, on top of your foundation, mixed with foundation, with eyeshadows, we could go on...

HOW TO CONTOUR

L.P.D. Definitively, this is it. You're welcome!

1. After applying your base products, take your bronzer. Using a large blusher brush, preferably one with a contoured tip as this will apply the product where you want it to go, start at the centre of the forehead and sweep down in a figure of '3', either side of the face. From the forehead, under the cheekbones, and under the jaw line. These points, when bronzed, help to add definition and structure to your face as the deep tone of the bronzer acts like a shadow.

2. Don't forget your neck. There's nothing worse than your face and neck looking two different shades. Sweep the excess bronzer down the neck, and along the décolletage if wearing a top that shows it.

3. Now for the highlighter. If using a cream product, pat on with your fingers. If using a powder, stick with a small brush. Apply on the cheekbones, down the centre of the nose and on the cupid's bow. These are the high points that the sun naturally hits. I also love to put a small amount on the apples of the cheeks for a subtle glow every time you smile.

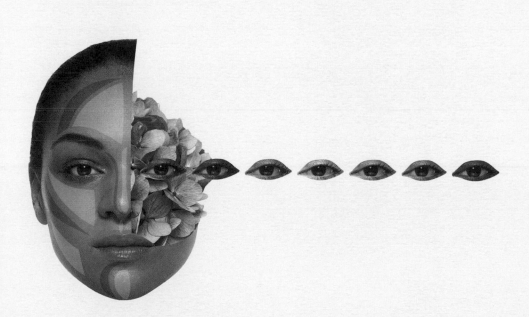

YOUR LIPS

IMPORTANT BECAUSE

THEY'RE THE FIRST THING THAT SOMEONE LOOKS AT IF THEY'RE ATTRACTED TO YOU.

THEY HAVE THE POWER TO BRIGHTEN OR DRAIN YOUR COMPLEXION.

YOU CAN CHEAT THEIR SIZE (WITHOUT NEEDLES).

CREATE A LIP ROUTINE

Avoid ruining any lipstick look by banishing dry lips first. This is a simple routine that you should be doing regularly.

HOW TO TAKE CARE OF LIPS

1. Exfoliate gently twice a week (mix a tiny amount of brown sugar with honey for the best DIY scrub).
2. Nourish lips with a hydrating or reparative balm (not petroleum-based) – this will help solve and protect any issues from cold, wind, chafing, you name it!
3. Don't forget SPF. The skin on your lips is thinner than on other parts of your face and body, and sensitive to UVA (photoageing) and UVB (sunburning) rays, so protect them all year round with an SPF lip balm.

COLOUR

You're going to want to find your happy place with a lip colour. In our opinion, red lipstick is right even when it's wrong (it's Sophie's trademark colour btw), but nailing it requires properly knowing your skin tone.

HOW TO PICK A LIP COLOUR

• Establish whether your basic complexion is light, medium or dark – quite self-explanatory.
• Understand your undertone. The easiest way is to look at the veins on the inside of your wrist in natural light. If they look green then your undertone is warm (yellow), if they're purple or blue you're cool (pink), and if you can't tell, you're either neutral or you're not very good at this game, in which case go to a beauty hall and ask a professional – they're very helpful!
• Now you can pick your colour. Stick to the tones you've identified, but pick anywhere on the spectrum from deep and dark reds to fluro colour.

For cool undertones
Go for blue-reds to balance out the pink (try Ruby Woo by MAC).

For warm undertones
Orange-reds complement warmer skin tones (try Rouge Allure Velvet in First Light by Chanel).

For neutral/olive undertones
Bright/true-reds look great on neutral skin tones (try Rouge Velvet The Lipstick in Rubi's Cute by Bourjois).

THE FITZPATRICK SCALE

Type 1: Light, Pale White	Blue-based and coral-toned reds – Maybelline Color Sensational Matte in Craving Coral.
Type 2: White, Fair	Blue/red shades – Christian Dior Rouge Dior Lip Colour in 999.
Type 3: Medium, White to Olive	Reds with a coral or orange base – MAC Lady Danger.
Type 4: Olive, Moderate Brown	Orange-toned and plum-based reds – YSL Rouge Pur Couture in Le Orange.
Type 5: Brown, Dark Brown	Full-on deep reds with blue undertones – Bobbi Brown Creamy Matte Lip Color in Red Carpet.
Type 6: Black, Very Dark Brown to Black	The deepest blue/red – Pat McGrath Mattetrance Lipstick in Elson.

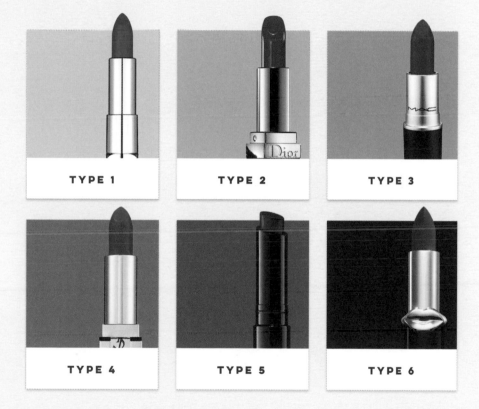

TYPE 1 TYPE 2 TYPE 3

TYPE 4 TYPE 5 TYPE 6

HOW TO DEFINE LIPS

1. Use a pencil that matches your natural lip colour to 'redraw' the shape of the lip you want before applying lipstick and fill in for extra-long-lasting wear.

2. Follow with lipstick. Apply some colour with a brush for precision and an even application. Straight-from-the-bullet is actually harder to get right.

3. Use a highlighter on the cupid's bow and in the centre of the lips for a three-dimensional finish.

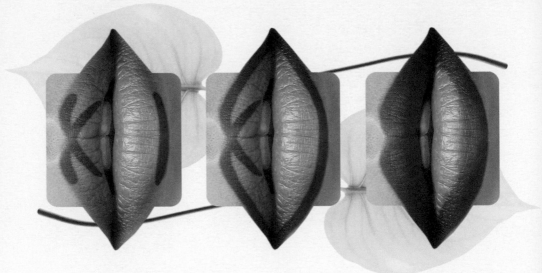

YOUR
HAIR

IMPORTANT BECAUSE

YOUR HAIR HAS THE POWER TO TRANSFORM YOUR LOOK MORE THAN ANY OTHER BEAUTY TRICK.

WE'VE ALL HAD DEVASTATING CUTS,
REGULAR BHDS (BAD HAIR DAYS),
OR A DIY COLOUR DISASTER.
HERE'S HOW TO HAVE ONLY GOOD HAIR DAYS
FROM NOW ON.

GREAT HAIR CHEATS

There are four pillars to creating good hair looks.

1. PREP

Like you'd prep your skin before makeup with moisturizer, primer, serums and masks, you need to prep your hair for the best finish, too.

L.P.D. I use a hair serum, because I find my hair is much shinier when I do, and who doesn't want glossy hair?! Serum also helps to nourish your scalp, which, in turn, gives you better, stronger hair. From someone who suffers from psoriasis, I can tell you, this is much needed.

S. B. Can I just tell you my flower bed analogy?

Go on then.

If you nourish the soil, the flowers will grow better. I'll leave you with that.

This comes from someone who has astro-turf in their back garden. My fave products are the OGX Nourishing Coconut Milk Anti-Breakage Serum and Onira Organics The Onira Oil. Both make my hair feel as silky as Sophie's cats. They are VERY silky.

I never use serum and tell hairdressers not to use it on me because it tends to wear my hair down. I get shine in my hair by heat styling, which means that I need to protect it first. So my prep is heat protection spray. Like SPF for your skin, it's so necessary. It creates a barrier around the hair cuticle to prevent heat from altering the strength and texture of your hair. My favourite is Percy & Reed The Perfect Blow Dry Makeover Spray. You can't over use it and it smells incredible.

OUR GOOD HAIR DAY TOP 5

Living Proof Perfect Hair Day Dry Shampoo	Means you only have to wash your hair once a week!
Larry King A Social Life For Your Hair	Just run it through all over for an expensive finished look.
Sam McKnight Cool Girl Barely There Texture Mist	Like the ultimate French girl texture in a can.
L'Oreal Elnett Hairspray	There is still no better, universally great hairspray.
Bumble & Bumble Brilliantine	The OG taming product that saves from frizz.

2. TEXTURE

We're not talking natural texture, we're talking putting in 'I just got out of bed and this is what I looked like, honest' texture (it definitely didn't). It's the secret to making your style look cool and effortless.

The truth. You have to take your natural texture out to put the cool texture in. Start smooth, then deconstruct by degrees. It's easier than it looks. Product is key. Here's how we do it.

> *L.P.D.* I like to use a dry shampoo. I can't remember life before it. Not only does it mean that I can get away with not washing my hair for a day longer, it also adds amazing texture and fragrance. My favourites are Colab Dry Shampoo because it smells incredible and adds the best texture. And Living Proof Perfect Hair Day Dry Shampoo. I love how lightweight this product is for a dry shampoo, and, again, it smells delish.

> *S.B.* I am a texture spray girl. It's the only styling product I use because my hair smooths really easily, but it needs some lift and grip to make it look cool. My favourites are Redken Wind Blown 05 Finishing Spray because it literally does what it says. As does my other favourite, Sam McKnight Cool Girl Barely There Texture Mist, enough said!

3. THE RIGHT TOOLS

For Waves

> *S.B.* I feel like I need to kick this one off, Lisa. I have discovered the holy grail of good hair. And this is no exaggeration. To everyone who messages me to ask about my amazing hair. Oh, if only you knew the truth. My hair is A DISASTER. Mousy, frizzy, broken, erratic. I could not DIY until I discovered this secret tool. It will legit change your life. (#notsponsored. But #shouldbe) (#jkng #butamI)

GHD Curve Classic Wave Wand

It's like a squashed version of a fat round tong. Why is this the secret? It gives the most amazing loose natural waves, rather than a ringlet curl, and it holds all day. With shine. What? We know.

> *L.P.D.* I have the complete opposite hair to Sophie. It's super thick, heavy and does not hold a curl. Soph curled my hair with it in a hotel in Paris once when we had five minutes to get ready, and since then I haven't looked back. Now I've cut my hair off short I rely on it even more. See what it looks like IRL on page 49.

For Smooth Hair

DAFNI Hair Straightening Brush

> Let me introduce you to DAFNI – also my nan's name – although Sophie has been calling the brush Betty (by mistake), until we typed this sentence and I corrected her. Literally a hairbrush that heats up and straightens your hair. No waiting around, no having to section your hair into 48 parts, you literally slowly brush your hair and it's smooth in seconds.

Warning: Think 'beauty experts' know everything? When Sophie first took this home she used it on wet hair ('I thought it was like a smoothing blowdry!') and clicked into consciousness when steam started coming off the roots. You DO have to dry your hair first.

It won't be poker straight but it's the perfect base for any styling afterwards. It's like a naturally smooth finish that makes you look put together at the very least.

Tangle Teezer

We are both obsessed with this cult product (but not as big of a fan as our prospective pets, who love to have their hair combed with this brush).

> My cat Coco has practically no hair, but she bloody loves a Tangle Teeze nonetheless, which just proves, it's super gentle even on half-bald, curly, skinny cats.

> If I start brushing my hair with it my dog Diddy will lie on his back so I have to brush him too.

This is the ultimate smoothing and detangling brush for wet hair, damaged hair, thick hair, coloured or permed hair, short hair, long hair, hair extensions, cat hair, dog hair.

Curly

> P.S. I bloody love Lee Stafford's Chopstick Styler.
> It literally transforms me into a Studio 54 dance queen.

4. ACCESSORIES

Embellishing your hair gives you the same impact as putting on a lipstick. It's easy, one step and show-stopping.

> *S.B.* If I smooth my hair and put it in a low pony tail, I'm not doing myself any favours. If I add a floppy velvet bow, it's suddenly a fashion statement that people stop me in the street to photograph (true story).

> *L.P.D.* Top knots are my go-to. If in doubt, chuck it up! The key to making it look like it took 30 minutes, rather than the 30-second reality, is to customize it. I'm obsessed with cool hair pins.

LISA LOVES: The Syd Pin by Syd Hayes – it's minimal, functional, industrial.

SOPHIE LOVES: An ASOS Oversized Velvet Bow – it's lady-like, elegant, extra.

SALON SPEAK

In the salon there are two languages: what you say and what a hairdresser says. For example:

> You: Hi, I'd like to have The Rachel from 1994 Friends.

> Hairdresser: She'd like to have the short to mid-length layered bob with feathered ends.

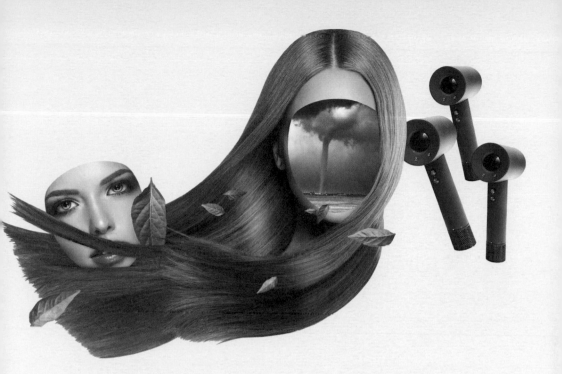

Understand how to speak hairdresser and you'll never leave a salon with a fake smile and murderous thoughts again. We've got some expert friends to give us the low-down.

CUTS WITH LARRY KING

You say: I want layers.

> Larry says: Eliminate bulk and create shape whilst keeping length, consider my hair texture to know what layering pattern will work best for my hair type, please.

You say: I want to look like Beyoncé.

> Larry's says: Here's a picture of Beyoncé, but I'll let you work with my hair texture and use your knowledge to adapt that photo to work best for me, thanks.

You say: I want a fringe.

Larry says: Only go as wide as my eyebrows so as not to open the face up too much, and remember the shorter the fringe the stronger the look.

You say: I had a fringe and now I don't want a fringe.

Larry says: Maybe I should consider having some well placed extensions to blend it out in the interim.

You say: I'd like a trim, please.

Larry says: Generally a trim is to maintain hair health, so I'll trust that you will cut off only what you think is really necessary to keep it looking tip top.

STYLE WITH SYD HAYES

You say: Beachy waves.

Syd says: Keep the barrel of a 25mm tong flat on top of the hair and twist leaving about 3cm out from the end to stop it bouncing back into a curl and keep it feeling loose.

You say: Dishevelled updo.

Syd says: Think what would Kate Moss do? Start with texture and ensure there is a grit and a plump feel to the hair. Lift the roots with thickening spray, only add volume where needed and pull out random sections around the ears to soften.

You say: Volume, please.

Syd says: Use a classic hot roller set and a thickening spray. Make sure the rollers sit on top of the section of hair so that the roller is tight and it does not drop. Only backcomb to add volume where it is needed, backcomb at the root only.

You say: Hollywood glam.

Syd says: A deep side part with a full set of uniformed curls, pinning to set the curl. At the front of the head make sure there is no root drag creating maximum root lift. Brush out when completely cool.

COLOUR WITH ADAM REED

You say: I think I'd like balayage please.

Adam says: A freehand colour technique using pre-lightener to lift the colour in pieces to totally and subtly enhance the natural colour of your hair.

You say: I think I'd like ombre please.

Adam says: A perfectly tonal seamless colour blend from root to finish, reducing in depth as you get to the ends.

You say: I'd like a dip dye please.

Adam says: A prominent tonal difference between roots and ends, literally as if hair has been dipped in colour.

You say: Highlights please! All over.

Adam says: Lightening the hair by placing colour throughout, but using a foil for a more precise placement. Lowlights add depth to the hair by using the same technique.

You say: I'd like to warm up my colour.

Adam says: What you think is warm, we might consider cool. In hairdresser terms...

WHAT ARE 'WARM TONES'?

Golden, copper, chestnut, auburn, chocolate

WHAT ARE 'COOL TONES'?

Mahogany, burgundy, beige, ash, violet, mauve, black, cinnamon

OUR HAIR HEROES

We've asked our personal and trusted hairdressers how they do our hair. So if you should ever want A Lisa or A Sophie, here's what to ask for (along with this picture, if you like).

THE SOPHIE

Adam Reed has two salons in London, is excellent at cut AND colour, and is my friend. Lucky me! (And him, of course...)

> *S.B.* I keep a strong outline using a traditional shear, then forward graduate throughout the front section in a concave to create a soft bevel without thinning the ends. Add invisible layers every third visit to add dimension. The colour is a mix of tones coined 'French cinnamon' with freehand beige cream in the front, away from the root.

THE LISA

Mathieu Clabaux has done my hair for four years, I never even ask him what to do, I just let him do his thing and it always looks amazing.

> *L. P. D.* I go for a long, concave bob with angled layers at the back to bring the weight to the front. Enhanced with light caramel balayage.

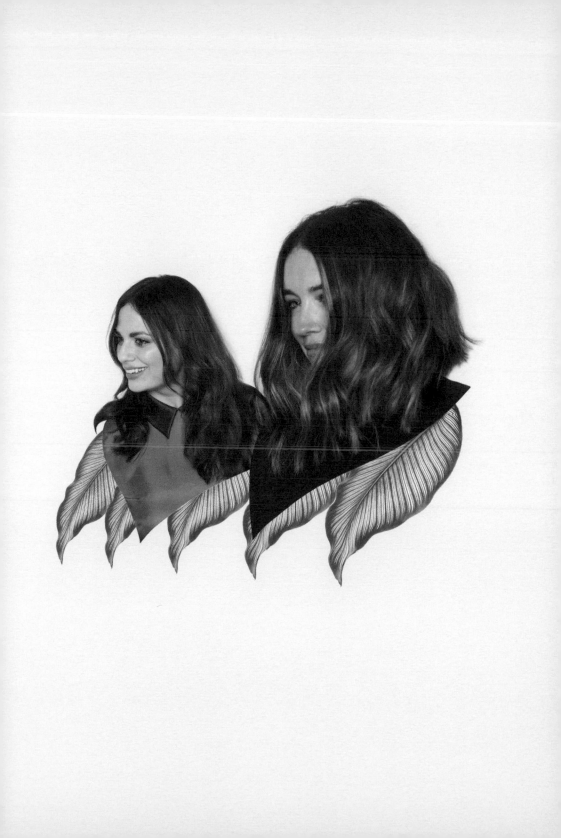

COLOUR

IMPORTANT BECAUSE

COLOUR IS EMOTIVE AND EFFECTIVE IN MANY WAYS.

AKA MAKEUP IS MEDICINE.

TURN TO THE PAGE THAT TALKS TO YOU THE MOST, THEN WEAR IT ON YOUR FACE TO FEEL GREAT.

SOMETIMES, THIS THEORY IS REFERRED TO AS 'CHROMOTHERAPY' – BUT IT'S SUPER SIMPLE, SO LET'S JUST CALL IT 'COLOUR'.

TURN TO THE PAGE THAT TALKS TO YOU THE MOST, THEN WEAR IT ON YOUR FACE TO FEEL GREAT.

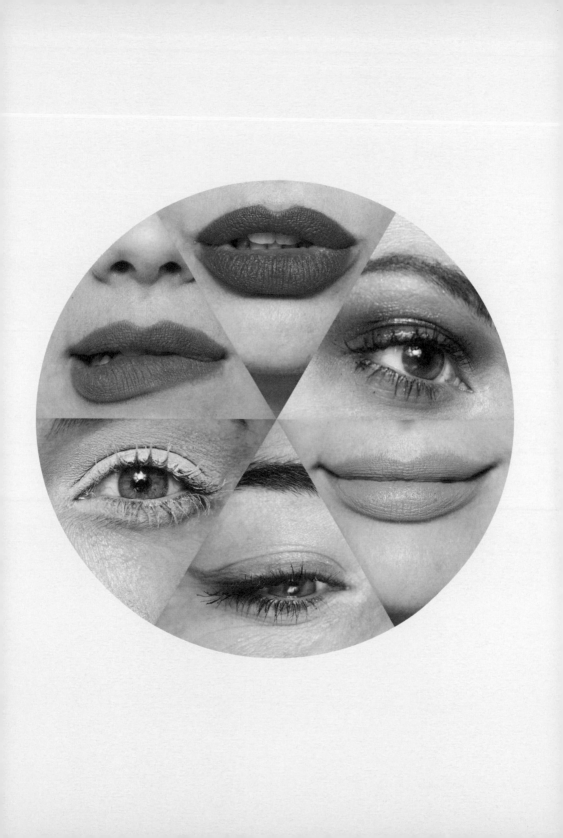

RED REPRESENTS

PHYSICAL ENERGY

VITALITY

STAMINA

GROUNDING

SPONTANEITY

STABILITY

PASSION

ORANGE REPRESENTS

CREATIVITY

PRODUCTIVITY

PLEASURE

OPTIMISM

ENTHUSIASM

EMOTIONAL EXPRESSION

YELLOW REPRESENTS

FUN

HUMOUR

LIGHTNESS

PERSONAL POWER

INTELLECT

LOGIC

CREATIVITY

GREEN REPRESENTS

BALANCE

HARMONY

LOVE

COMMUNICATION

SOCIABILITY

NATURE

ACCEPTANCE

BLUE REPRESENTS

CALMNESS

PEACE

LOVE

HONESTY

KINDNESS

TRUTH

INNER PEACE

EMOTIONAL DEPTH

DEVOTION

VIOLET REPRESENTS

INTUITION
IMAGINATION

UNIVERSAL FLOW

MEDITATION

ARTISTIC QUALITIES

BEAUTY TOOLS

IMPORTANT BECAUSE

COME ON NOW, WHERE HAVE YOU BEEN?

IF YOU WANT THE BEST RESULTS,
YOU NEED THE RIGHT TOOLS.

BRUSHES ARE YOUR BEST TOOLS.
IN FACT, THIS PAGE SHOULD BE CALLED BRUSHES.

BRUSHES

> *S.B.* I've got over 300 makeup brushes, I can't just put 5, can I put brands instead? Because cotton buds are a good one too. The wooden ones. #savetheplanet. OK fine, 5. Here goes.

SOPHIE'S TOP 5

Zoeva Concealer Brush	It's my secret weapon for a smoky eye. Yes, eyes! Rule breaker.
Charlotte Tilbury Powder & Sculpt Brush	Perfect for dispensing not too much and not too little.
bareMinerals Original Powder Foundation Brush	This is my mirror-free, buff-it-all-over, lazy but perfect approach to foundation.
MAC 316 Lip Brush	For concealer. I know I know, but the flat head lets you pat on the right amount of product.
Benefit Angled Brow Brush and Spoolie	Just brushing your brows up after makes them look fuller. I cannot do my brows without this.

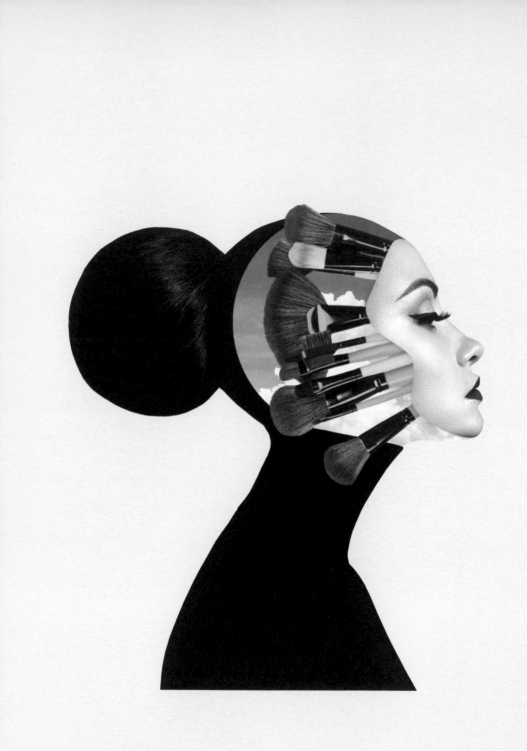

LISA'S TOP 5

Beautyblender	Always dampen it to stop the product soaking in. It's the BEST tool for foundation because it gives such an even, beautiful finish.
Crown Eye Brush C163	The small head is so brilliant for blending under eyes or for creating a smoky liner.
Wayne Goss Brush 10 Cheek Brush	Tapered so amazing for bronzing, highlighting and blusher.
Real Techniques PowderBleu Soft Shadow Brush	Amazing for blending to give the perfect airbrushed smoky eye.
Louise Constad Lip Brush	Super flat, which means you can get the perfect precise pout.

OTHER ESSENTIAL TOOLS

- Dual pencil sharpener.
- Pointed tweezers.
- Cute makeup bag.
- Lash curlers.
- Lash glue.

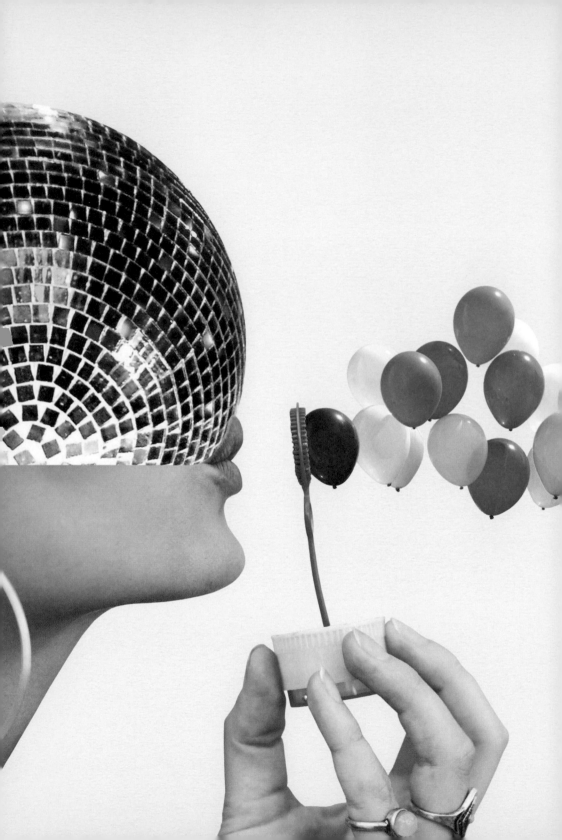

FOR THE GOOD TIMES

FOR THE GOOD TIMES, THE BEST TIMES,
THE TIMES YOU REMEMBER, ANYTIME,
AND EVERY TIME. ALL THE BEAUTY IDEAS AND
ADVICE YOU'D NEED FOR ANY OCCASION.

GOING
OUT

YOU WILL HAVE DIFFERENT BEAUTY
REQUIREMENTS DEPENDING ON WHO
YOU ARE GOING OUT WITH,
WHERE YOU ARE GOING,
WHAT YOUR 'GOING OUT' INVOLVES.
THE TRICK IS TO LAYER AND BUILD
YOUR LOOK TO FIT THE INTENSITY
OF YOUR EVENING. THE CHOICE IS YOURS,
BUT CONSIDER THIS YOUR STARTING BLOCK.
ON YOUR MARKS, GET SET, GO OUT.

FOOD

S.B. Oh god, the number of times I've eaten a burrito and forgotten I'm wearing lipstick until someone surreptitiously wipes my chin with the napkin.
#girlcode

L.P.D. What about when you've spent hours doing your makeup and they dim the lights till you're just candlelit. What a waste.

Food obviously means eating will be involved, so don't bother with lip colour. No one wants to see lipstick transference or monotonous reapplication. Instead, make it all about the eyes.

Shimmer looks are the best subtle makeup in all light, because it catches the light.

EYESHADOW DECISIONS

Liquid metallic shimmer	More of a mirror finish. The most dramatic option. Easy to blend and looks great all over the lid or just in the centre of the eye.
Cream shimmer shadow	More subtle than metallic. Hundreds of shades to choose from. Gives a wet-look finish. Looks great in a nude or a bold.
Powder shimmer shadow	Pat on with your fingers for a low-key, subtle finish. Apply with a wet brush if you really want to make the most of it.

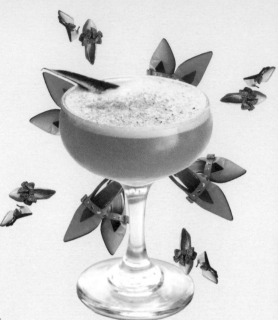

COCKTAILS

L.P.D. I love a cocktail. My 3 favourites have to be Aperol spritz, Amaretto sour and a frozen strawberry daiquiri.

S.B. I cannot drink cocktails because I am a control freak. I can measure my drunkenness by the state of my eyeliner, and trust me, it's not pretty after any amount of tequila.

You have the low-light-appropriate shimmer base. Now up the ante with eyeliner to build and define your look.

LISA LOVES: Jet black kohl liner in the waterline and smudged below the lashes, because it looks better the more it moves, so it's not a concern no matter how many cocktails happen.

SOPHIE LOVES: Defining her look with a sharp feline flick tapered out from inner to outer corner. It doesn't always have to be black, a coloured liner is a little more relaxed and can say more about you than you even know. Check page 50.

CHEEKS

Add highlighter to refresh your face. It will wake your whole complexion up, but is also attention-grabbing in the most subtle way possible.

LIPS

Well, we're assuming they'll be busy hugging the side of your cocktail glass. Stick to a stain that will settle into your lips rather than imprint onto your drink. Although, a lipstick mark is a good way of identifying to whom on the table that espresso martini belongs...

THE PERFECT APEROL SPRITZ 3-2-1 RECIPE

Fill a wine glass with ice and add:
• 3 parts prosecco
• 2 parts Aperol
• 1 part soda water
Mix, add slice of orange, consume responsibly.

OUT OUT

S.B. What is out out exactly?

L.P.D. For me? It's a bar until it closes, then probably a hip hop club and dancing till that closes. Then getting chips and cheese on the way home. What's yours?

Um. Getting dinner after the cinema instead of before?

If this is the ultimate night out, it needs the ultimate eye makeup (we're still assuming you're using your lips to drink/eat/talk/sing/kiss/whatever).

EYES

Build. It. Up. There will never be a better time than now to pile on the glitter. Whether you layer it over a smoky eye, or wear it by itself, glitter makes everything extra. (Extra special.)

SOPHIE LOVES: Putting a dot of liquid glitter under the bottom lashes for an easy but low-maintenance impact.

HOW TO DO LOW-DEF GLITTER

1. Take a flat lipstick brush, dab it in your chosen glitter shadow (Stila Magnificent Metals Glitter & Glow Liquid Eyeshadow or Hourglass Scattered Light Glitter Eyeshadow are both great ready-to-go products).
2. Apply below the lashes in the middle only.
3. Finish with mascara.

LISA LOVES: Showering in the stuff. She covers the entire lid from the socket line down to the lash line in a combination of glitter colours – particularly high-impact jewel tones.

HOW TO DO HIGH-DEF GLITTER

1. Put a glitter glue on first.
2. Pat the glitter pigment on (try Karla Cosmetics Glitter or EcoStardust Biodegradable Glitter) with a flat concealer brush.
3. Layer until you can layer no more.
4. Add tonnes of mascara instead of faux lashes for a cool look.

LISA-APPROVED BEST GLITTER GLUE: Paintglow Glitter Gel – it's super cheap and available online.

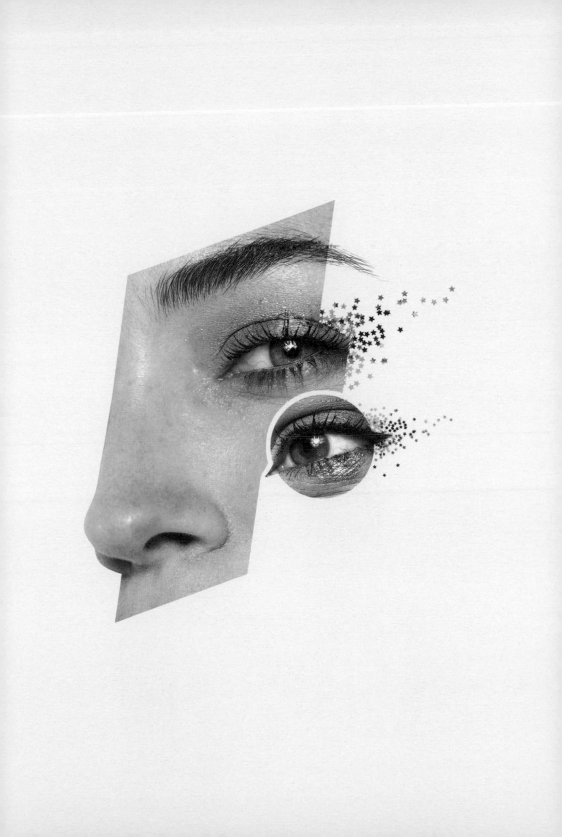

STAYING IN

…IS THE NEW GOING OUT, DEPENDING ON WHO YOU
LISTEN TO. LISTEN TO US; IT'S WONDERFUL FOR VERY
MANY REASONS, INCLUDING BUT NOT EXCLUSIVE TO
SECRETLY CRAWLING TO BED WHILE EVERYONE WORRIES
ABOUT HOW MANY UBERS ARE AVAILABLE IN YOUR NECK
OF THE WOODS. IT'S CALLED A FRENCH EXIT AND IT'S
YOUR REWARD FOR COOKING DINNER. YOU'RE WELCOME

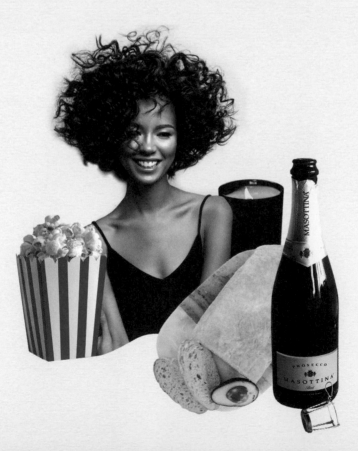

DINNER PARTIES

We're talking about throwing them, not going to them. As such, dinner parties can be stressful. How many people are coming? Oh my god how many courses are you doing? When the hell are you going to get ready? Just like you prep your ingredients think about prepping your outfit and makeup look too. It'll save you spinning out.

> *I. P.D.* Keep it simple, because from my vast experience...

> *S.B.* Yep, you are never not throwing a party.

> ...cooking always takes longer than you think. I can do my whole face in two minutes. But then it is my job.

> I sweat my makeup off cos of the hob so I have to chuck lipstick on when the doorbell goes.

QUICK FIXES TO STOP YOUR MAKEUP MELTING OFF

• Use a lip and cheek tint rather than a cream or powder because it will sink in and stay there. So when you're wiping tomato sauce off your cheek, you won't take your makeup with you.
• Prep with primer and set makeup with a translucent powder to help prevent too much sweat shine and base movement.
• Put your lipstick and perfume next to the door with a mirror, so you can literally apply it when the bell goes. Also handily masks the scent of cooking fat in the hallway.
• Water-resistant mascara. Cooking almost always starts with chopping onions. No one wants black teardrops on their mashed potatoes.
• Top off whatever product you've used to shape and define your brows with a clear waterproof gel. You can even do that in the morning knowing they're not going to move all day.
• VITAL: Always have a glass of prosecco on hand to keep your mood calmer than your hair is looking.

• Oh yeah, hair. Don't even worry about it. Cheating is the answer. This is where chucking it up and adding an accessory is absolutely exactly the right thing to do (see page 44).

SOPHIE'S 'INTERNET-BREAKING' CAMEMBERT TEAR 'N' SHARE

• coarse polenta
• pre-made pizza dough. Or make your own, but it won't be as good and who has the time?
• boxed Camembert
• beaten egg
• poppy seeds
• sesame seeds
• fresh rosemary
• garlic

1. Line a very big, high-sided baking tray with greaseproof paper and scatter polenta in it.
2. Tear and roll your pizza dough into walnut-sized balls and put aside.
3. Place boxed Camembert in the middle of the tray, dip the dough balls in beaten egg, then dip into the seeds, alternating between poppy, sesame or plain, and place around the cheese, leaving a little space in-between.
4. Set aside for an hour to prove; everything should all join up.
5. Take the Camembert out of the box, cut a disc from the top and stab rosemary and garlic slices randomly into the cheese.
6. Remove the box from the dough ball tray and put the now-naked cheese back in its place.
7. Drizzle with oil and bake at 180°C/350°F/gas 4 for 25 minutes.
8. Tear and share, but the share part is optional.

LISA'S PEOPLE-PLEASING EASY TRUFFLE PASTA

• mushrooms (optional)
• garlic
• fresh pasta
• truffle butter
• truffle oil (the good stuff)
• salt and pepper
• Parmesan (absolutely loads)

1. Slice the mushrooms (if using) and sauté with garlic for approximately 10 minutes in a saucepan.
2. Boil the pasta for approximately 4–6 minutes – don't overdo it.
3. Drain the pasta, put it back in the pan and immediately stir in a big teaspoon of the truffle butter, followed by lashings of truffle oil. I like a lot!
4. Add the mushrooms, a pinch of salt, pepper to taste and serve into bowls.
5. Finish with shaved Parmesan, at least a handful per person.
6. Eat, enjoy and definitely lick the bowl.

LOVE

YOU KNOW IT'S THE REAL THING WHEN
MAKEUP DOESN'T EVEN COME INTO
THE EQUATION ANYMORE. BUT WE'RE TALKING
BEFORE THAT; THE RELATIONSHIP BETWEEN
MAKEUP AND DATING. WHETHER IT'S
TRANSFORMATIVE OR JUST AN
EMPOWERING BOOST TO BUILD YOUR CONFIDENCE.
WHEN YOU WANT TO FEEL YOUR
MOST ATTRACTIVE, YOUR MAKEUP BAG CAN HELP.

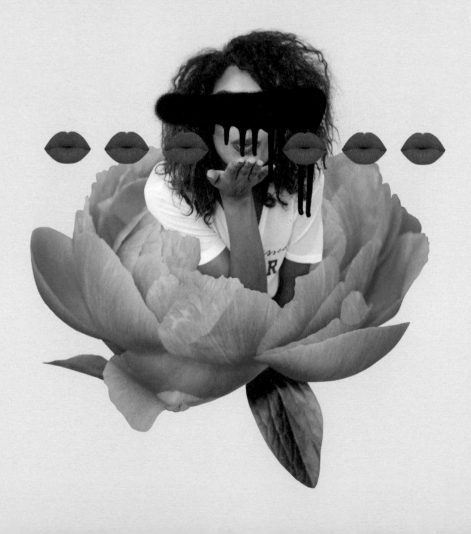

FIRST DATE

L.P.D. Don't wear lipstick or gloss cos of the kissing.

S.B. No! You don't kiss on the first date.

Yes you're right, wear lipstick – it'll be like a barrier. (I think on my first dates I've always kissed though.)

whispers Yeah. Me too.

We're talking first impressions here, so who do you want to be? YOU is the answer, if YOU is all bold brows and contour then please, please, stick to the formula, because if you present yourself as someone else, this relationship ain't going anywhere. What we suggest is you, but better.

BROWS

Defined equals strong. Groomed brows make you look like you care about yourself, and therefore someone else should care about you, too.

EYES

A smoky liner is less maintenance and impact than a hard liquid line, but does all the eye-emphasizing you need. It's also easy to achieve. Just take a kohl liner, draw along your lash line – don't worry if it's a bit wonky. And then blend with a 'pencil brush'. Suddenly you're Kate Moss in 1994 without even trying.

LIPS

Important. The laws of attraction state that your date will be looking at your lips.

WHAT YOUR FIRST DATE LIPS SAY ABOUT YOU

Red	Bold, confident and passionate. It's sexy, innit?
Pink	Innocent and creative. It's the fun factor.
Burgundy	Strong and decisive, maybe a little hard to get with a dark side.
Coral	Enthusiastic and playful, you're approachable and warm.
Nude	You've nothing to hide and a lot to give.

BLIND/DATING APP DATE

L.P.D. I've never had a blind date or used a dating app.

S.B. Oh my god, I have. He told me he lived in a magical land called Leatherhead and said my head was so big it wouldn't fit through the door. I utilised my emergency exit strategy – aka a text resulting in my sister rescuing me from the bar.

Leatherhead is near where I live and it's definitely not magical.

The person you are meeting is most likely as nervous as you are, and you both have little expectation. Be approachable. We consulted our single friends – the consensus was 'less is more'.

SKIN

Don't: Cake it on. It will knock out all your contours and your own glow won't show.
Do: Mix liquid foundation with a drop of highlighter and apply with a damp Beautyblender for a seamless, natural finish.

CONCEALER

Don't: Layer concealer and powder. It will gather in the creases and do more emphasizing than concealing.
Do: Brighten under your eyes with a liquid one shade lighter than your complexion, to draw attention.

EYES

Don't: Go full-on. What if you go to a dark bar and your smoky eye looks like an endless black hole?
Do: Use highlighter in the centre of your eyes to brighten and go for a lengthening jet black mascara to make the most of your lashes and open your eyes.

LIPS

Don't: Go overboard. What if it's on your teeth? What if it transfers to your prosecco glass and then the bridge of your nose?
Do: A nude gloss with a hint of pink or coral to add a hit of colour and health. Make it an aside, not a statement.

Actually, do dodge the lipstick. You don't want to ever be worrying about how you look.

> I had a contact lens reaction and had to wear glasses for a while which totally knocked my confidence. My mum told me to accept a date with this guy who had been chasing me and who I wasn't that interested in, just to test it out. I went with glasses, he fancied me anyway, I felt great and we dated for a few months (before he turned out to be a total idiot). Moral of the story is, glasses are sexy.

THIRD DATE (*RAISES EYEBROWS*)

S.B. Obviously, we're not dictating the third date rule. It might be seventeenth, it might be first, but basically, we want to talk about sex makeup.

L.P.D. This is a hard one. Personally, in that scenario makeup is the furthest thing from my mind.

Are you kidding? Personally I think about what I'm going to look like in the morning.

IF YOU'RE SOPHIE:

You want to wake up looking naturally beautiful. This involves subtle pre-planning, and it looks like this...
• Tinted lashes: So they're still defined once you've taken your mascara off, and there will be no chance of smudging on the pillow.
• Groomed brows: Not with makeup, with wax and tint so they're pretty much perfect without any effort.
• Treatment foundation: There are some you can wear overnight that let your skin breathe whilst giving you a light coverage.

IF YOU'RE LISA:

Makeup-wise, you'll only worry about the issues that resulted from the night before...
• Lip balm: Dry lips happen. Always carry a nourishing balm that will replenish what was snogged off.
• Natural sheen: Put some highlighter on the apples of your cheeks for a natural-looking 'well exercised' glow. Ahem.
• Redness corrector: Stubble rash is a b!tch. Have a multi-tasking concealer in your bag with nourishing serum that will both cool and conceal.

EMERGENCY LOVE KIT:

- Charlotte Tilbury Magic Away Liquid Concealer.
- bareMinerals Pure Transformation Night Treatment.
- Gatineau Perfection Ultime Nourishing Lip Balm.
- Benefit High Beam.

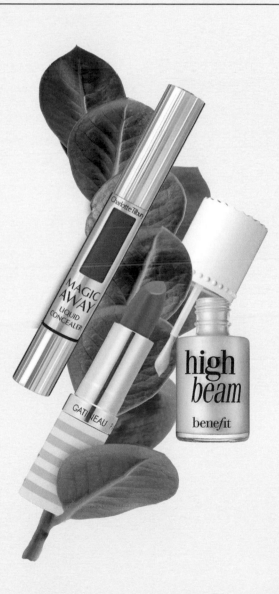

WEDDING

THE ONE DAY YOU WILL MOST AGONISE
OVER THE STATE OF YOUR FACE,
AND RIGHTLY SO.

WHETHER YOU'RE THE BRIDE,
THE MOTHER OF THE BRIDE, PART OF
THE WEDDING PARTY OR EVEN A GUEST,
WEDDINGS BRING OUT THE BEAUTY
OBSESSIVE IN ALL OF US.

WE'VE BOTH HAD ONE, WE'VE BOTH BEEN TO
THOUSANDS (OK, APPROXIMATELY 70 BETWEEN US),
LISA EVEN HAS BRIDE MAKEUP
RESPONSIBILITY SOMETIMES (GOOD
FRIENDS ONLY) SO WE COME WITH EXPERIENCE.

BRIDE

This is the only checklist you need.

☐ PREP

Do you want a spray tan, lashes, brow shape and tint? If so, do a dry run first. The hen do is the perfect time to test if lash extensions looks more camel than cute.

☐ INSPIRATION

Take some reference pictures, but be realistic – no one can transform you into Giselle, but your other half doesn't want to marry her anyway – this is about letting your makeup artist understand in what direction you want to go.

☐ TRIAL

Do it MAX 4 weeks in advance. You want your skin to be the same as it will on the big day. There is no point trialling with a tan that won't be there in a few months.

☐ TRUST

Be guided by your makeup artist, but don't let them take control. You know what suits you, what you like and what you feel most beautiful in.

☐ PLAN

Wear a top that is a similar colour to your dress to give you the most realistic approximation of your wedding day.

☐ AVOID

Trend-led makeup looks. Stick with classics. You've got to look at these photos forever. This doesn't mean in the evening you can't chuck on a bright orange lip or a touch of glitter for the party, but don't risk something you might be embarrassed by in a few years. Just count yourself lucky you're not getting married in the 80s.

☐ GLOW

This is your wedding day buzz word. Matte makeup might look good in the mirror but not so much in daylight or pictures. Keeping the highlight in the right place is key.
• Glowy primer under foundation (recommend BECCA Backlight Priming Filter).
• Dewy, longwear, liquid foundation (recommend Benefit Hello Happy Soft Blur Foundation).
• Powder or liquid highlighter on the high points of your face (see below).
• Add a flush of colour to the apples of your cheeks. A glowing complexion isn't just about highlighter, it's about looking healthy.

☐ PHOTOS

There will be flash at some point – use it to your advantage:
• DO add highlighter on your cheekbones, cupids bow and a small amount down the centre of your nose for extra glowiness (and shoulders and collarbone if your dress is strapless).
• DO NOT let anyone come near you with a highlighting concealer under your eyes. Your photos will be RUINED. Trust us.

☐ DELEGATE

Make sure your bridesmaid has your lipstick and anti-shine powder on hand for top ups throughout the day. It doesn't matter if her phone now doesn't fit in her bag. This is your day.

BRIDESMAIDS

First off, this day may not be about you, but still, you do want to look nice. However, if you have an idea about wearing something bold like a red lip, run it by the bride first. You're going to be in the pictures, so you want to have beautiful fresh skin – see bride's checklist. Also...

• Avoid strip lashes – bridesmaids are usually the first to cry and the last on the dance floor. You don't want to be worrying about losing them. Likewise, use a water-resistant mascara.

• Neutral tones are great, because you can build them up to the max, but they still look understated, aka respectful to the bride.

• Avoid blusher that has too much red in it – you'll be running around like a headless chicken doing your bridesmaid duties. Your natural colour will come through – stick to coral and pink tones, it will enhance but not overpower your complexion.

A LETTER FROM LISA ABOUT TIMINGS

Dear readers, when I do friends' weddings, I never do the bride first. I always start with the mother of the bride, because she's often most anxious about what she'll look like – but also the one who annoys the bride the most, so the sooner she's glammed and out the room the better. Next up, depending on the number of bridesmaids, I'll get at least one done. (Though usually I ask them to do their own, because these days brides have loads. I had seven, so can't really talk.) The bride's makeup should be started two hours before they need to leave, ready to go one hour before, allowing time to settle and final touches to be added. Love Lisa x

P.S. if you are the makeup artist, you'll always signal the arrival of the bride by walking into the ceremony just before she does. The amount of times I've had 120 people stand up and gasp when I walk in, then groan when they realise I'm not the bride.

M.O.B. AKA MOTHER OF THE BRIDE

Hi parents. Please listen to the makeup artist. You might usually wear makeup, you might not, but let the makeup artist work their magic. Tell them if you want it natural, that's fine, but trust them. Relinquish control. You'll be in photos, this is a special moment for you. You need eyebrows.

Treat yourself. This is a very special day for you, and you'll want to look amazing. So focus on the following tricks...

BROWS

Maybe the most important youthful makeup trick. As we age we lose definition in our bone structure and features, but honestly, drawing in and defining eyebrows helps restore it. If you don't have a tail to your brow, fill it in (see page 20). It lifts your cheekbones and opens your eyes.

LIPS

If you've lost volume in your lips, you can add the definition that's disappeared using a nude lip liner the same colour as your lips. Make the nib sharp, and carefully trace your natural outline, even taking it out a little on the cupids bow area, then fill in. Go over the top with your chosen lipstick – satin finish will be the most plumping and will stay put for longer – blot, repeat.

BASE

A heavy, high-coverage foundation might be tempting, but it's also quite ageing. Instead, use a dewy liquid foundation and then conceal over any pigmentation or imperfections that show through afterwards. It's a more natural, fresh and youthful trick.

FYI: Everyone can do their own makeup – especially if you have this book and like to practise. So, if you're determined to do one thing professionally, make it your hair. Much harder to get right on your own.

WEDDING GUEST

Take into consideration the time of year, the type of wedding and the venue. There are so many variables when it comes to being a guest. Here are a few of our own experiences.

SOPHIE AT THE SOUTH OF FRANCE WEDDING OF JOELY AND JAMES

I went for taupe glitter smoke and orange lip. Punchy, I know, but I knew the sun would be high, the guest list super stylish, and my blue Erdem dress was so incredible that it needed dramatic daytime makeup to set it off.

LISA AT THE MARRAKECH WEDDING OF LAURA AND SAMUELE

The most incredible, beautiful, eclectic venue (El Fenn – google it). The vibe was cool, fun and colourful. So I matched my lipstick to my fave wall in the hotel, paired it with groomed curls and a spangly Matthew Williamson chain mail dress.

SOPHIE AT THE INDIAN CITY WEDDING OF SEETA AND BHAV

As a family member, I went all out with the outfit, but I also knew a lot of the guests would be more understated, so I didn't want to look attention grabbing. I kept my makeup low key with feline flick eyeliner that complemented the theme, but let the accessories do the talking

LISA AT THE SUBURBAN TIPI TENT WEDDING OF HELEN AND ED

A field transformed into a glittery world of joy. I wanted an outfit to match, so wore blue sequinned trousers with a black top. Hair was down, textured and boho, and makeup with layers of glitter shadow paired with natural skin, so that I didn't have to worry about my base moving in the heat.

SOPHIE AT THE CORNISH BEACH WEDDING OF JON AND LAURA

Windy beach, fifteen minute walk to the field reception, super cool, bohemian and bloody beautiful. I wore sneakers with my dress, and a bold red lipstick with my messy hair. Balanced and low maintenance.

LISA AT THE LONDON PUB NYE WEDDING OF KYRA AND DAN

Awesome London experience, from the red bus transport to the Hackney pub venue. I went for an accessorized top knot, as I knew this would be the type of wedding where you'd be dancing from start to finish. Paired it with eyeliner flicks for an Amy Winehouse vibe.

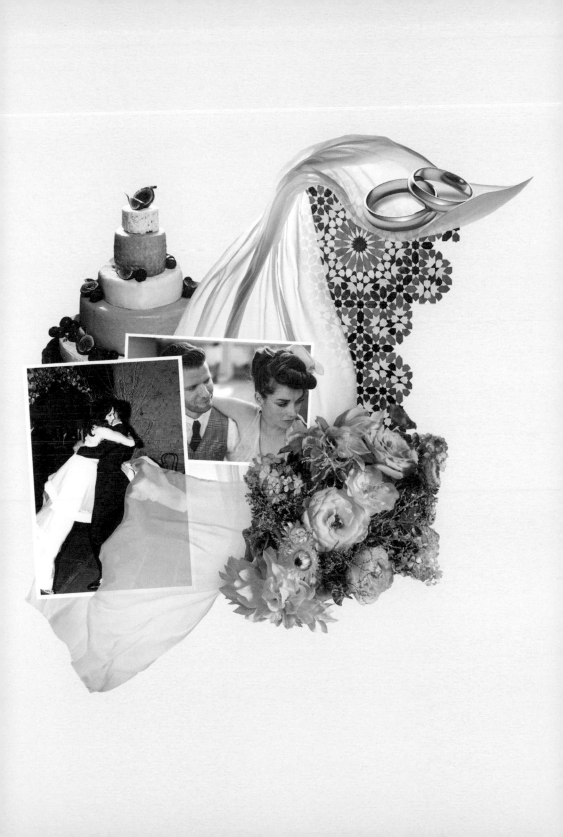

GIVING BIRTH

WE CURRENTLY DON'T HAVE A BABY
BETWEEN US (EXCEPTING THE FURRY KIND),
SO WE TESTED OUR THEORIES ON
OUR FRIENDS WHO DO. MORE ON THAT LATER.
YOU NEED TO ACCEPT THAT YOUR
ROUTINE IS GOING TO GO OUT THE WINDOW.
DO YOU CARE? IF SO READ ON,
IF NOT, SKIP TO THE NEXT CHAPTER.

BEFORE

This could be the last time you have some pamper time to yourself for a while, so if you're a 'groomer', plan ahead; book in your hair, nails, pedi, wax, whatever. Remember, the arrival of a baby is unpredictable, so book waaay ahead. If you don't think you're a groomer, treat yourself. We're not saying perfect nails is the answer, but this is valuable you time. You will want to retain a vestige of yourself, and this is a very easy way to do it.

⚡ Bianca Presto has joined the group

> 'The little f**ker came early so any prep went out the window. On the plus side, I was admitted straight from work, so I think I still had a face full of makeup four days later when she finally arrived.'

FYI: Officially no treatments can be done in the first trimester, just enjoy being pregnant for a bit first.

HAIR

We have it on good authority that you may go a year and a half before you see a salon again. Highlights, trim, glossing treatment, Brazilian blowdry, get the works. It will help you feel good once you're out the other side and might make you love your first baby pics even more, too.

TAN

If you're feeling at all self-conscious about your new body shape, stretch marks, etc (women do, it's natural, but you don't need us to tell you how amazing your body is for what it's doing right now), a tan can actually help.

There is a little black dress theory of tanning: In the same way an LBD is flattering, a darker tan diffuses the contrast of the shadows on your skin from cellulite or lumps or bumps, and it makes you look and feel healthier. It's why humans spend their holidays tanning on the beach, it's why we fake it all year round. Embrace it – but only in the second or third trimester.

NAILS

As short as you're comfortable with, because you'll be using your hands a lot and you want to be gentle. Try shellac. It doesn't chip, it dries instantly and it's that little bit of grooming perfection that makes you feel like you have your sh*t together even when you so don't.

Kyra White has joined the group

'I'm about to pop. One of my fears is that I won't have time to do my nails weekly as I have for the past 20 years. I'm sure there are more important things to be worried about at this stage, but each to their own.'

FACIAL/MASSAGE

Ah, that natural pregnancy glow. Some have it, some don't, but even those who do will suffer the hormonal skin-ravaging surges. Acne? Pigmentation? Sorry guys, just remember it's temporary, but a professional pregnancy facial can take the edge off.

Laura lou has joined the group

'As long as I leave looking "faux-fresh", even when I'm not feeling it, I've got my money's worth.'

You've been growing a person for the last few months, we think you've earned some indulgent alone time. A good pregnancy massage is a great way of naturally easing the ailments of being pregnant. It will improve circulation, tension, headaches, stress and anxiety, and give you better sleep so you'll be better prepared when the baby comes. And that natural glow we just mentioned? It'll go some way to boosting that, too.

BEST TRIED-AND-TESTED TREATMENTS

Cowshed Udderly Gorgeous Body	Gentle, so best for relaxing.
Elemis Peaceful Pregnancy Massage	Best for getting rid of muscle tension, aches and pains.

WAX

OK, here's the thing. Yeah yeah, you don't care, it's not about you, it's about your baby, blah blah. Only while you're giving birth, it's not even about you, it's about your vagina. The theory is a wax might hurt more because your body is producing extra blood and fluids, and that makes your skin more sensitive. If you care about what everyone in the room thinks about your grooming (you really shouldn't, they just want to get your baby out, but you're only human, so...), then man up. The birth will hurt more, but you'll be safe in the knowledge your pubes are immaculate. P.S. ever thought about a heart shape?

Bianca Presto has joined the group

> 'Turns out no-one cared about my fanny hair maintenance because: a) we had more important things to care about; and b) she came out the sunroof.'

DURING

First question; do you even bother?!

↳ *Lauren Murdoch-Smith has joined the group*

> 'I checked and reapplied my make up while I was in hospital, because I just wanted to feel a bit nicer. Ultimately you're not in control of anything else and you're leaving your dignity at the door.'

Ok then, so let's talk about birth makeup.

Let nature do its thing first. You are not going to need a blush; you're in the middle of the hardest 'workout' of your life. You're going to have a beautiful, natural flush.

If your brows and lashes are tinted, there's nothing else to think about, except...

We've given you some useful tips in The Disruptors. Turn to page 118, Rush Hour. Then see page 106, Crying. Just saying...

AFTER

Seriously? Go to sleep.

But actually, this is where makeup can come in really, really useful. It's that faux fresh thing, and if you can convince your reflection you're doing OK, you're halfway there.

Concealer will become your NBF, blusher will become your secret weapon.

A dot of blusher on the apples of your cheeks will bring your face back to life. You may feel like a zombie, but no zombie has glowing pink cheeks.

Eyebrows, just a one second swipe up and across with fibre gel will help lift your eye area and hold everything in place, plus you can do it one-handed.

Blue mascara. Like the blue particles in the washing powder you're now using 8 times a day, blue pigmented mascara has the same brightening and whitening effect on your tired eyes.

Keep a lip balm in your baby bag. Lack of sleep contributes to dehydrated lips, and this is, believe it or not, the one thing that can make you look the most tired and sickly. Simple, effective, true.

Jess Diner has joined the group

> 'I brought some mascara and concealer for the post-birth pictures because I didn't want to look at the snaps for the rest of time and think I looked like sh*t.'

WORK

YOU PLAN YOUR OUTFIT TO THE FINEST DETAIL,
YOUR MAKEUP SHOULD BE NO DIFFERENT.

YOU DO NOT NEED MAKEUP
TO BE POWERFUL, OR TO DO YOUR JOB.

BUT YOU CAN'T DENY THE CONFIDENCE-
BOOSTING POWERS OF IT.

YOUR PROFESSIONAL IMAGE
SHOULD NOT BE UNDERESTIMATED.

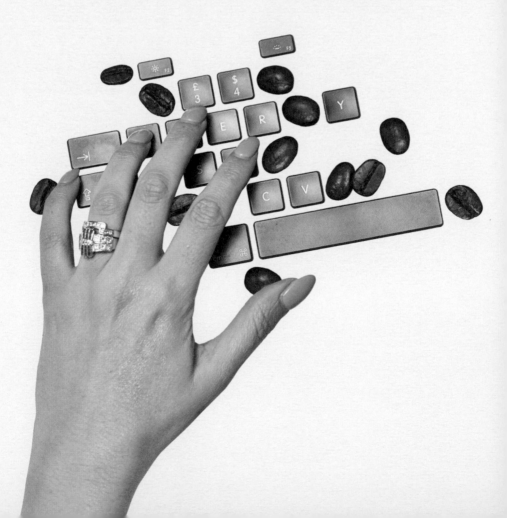

JOB INTERVIEW

If you want the job then you'll want to impress – obviously with your CV first, then your sparkling conversation, smart responses, exceptional experience. And then subliminally, your groomed appearance. Essentially, you're trying to be attractive to someone. Not romantically but professionally. Even so, some of the same ideas apply.

THE NO-NOS

It's amazing what prospective employees will notice without even noticing.

Chipped nails
You'll be presenting ideas, gesticulating while you talk, your hands are part of the show. Make them smart, neat and simple. Maybe even check Colour on page 50 for the secret message you want to convey.

Messy hair
Messy anything for that matter. We're not talking about texture here. You want to look like you've made an effort. A ponytail or a neat top knot is always a safe option.

Foundation tide mark
Check your makeup in natural light before you leave. A neck that doesn't match your face is not cool.

FIRST DAY

Just like your first day at school, it can be nerve-racking. You'll know what to do without us having to tell you. Think about your favourite ever item of clothing and how great it makes you feel when you wear it. What is your makeup equivalent of that? That will be your 'confident face'. Put it on immediately.

These people that you're about to meet are potentially going to become a big part of your life and maybe even good friends. Therefore it is important to be yourself from day one.

TIP: Don't underestimate the conversational power of makeup. If you've run out of things to say to the person next to you, ask them what their favourite Glossier product is. It's a bonding experience, trust us.

DO...

• Something like an eyeliner flick that looks smart and sassy at the same time. It hints at a bit of personality whilst still being work-appropriate.
• Embrace a bold lip. IF it makes you feel good. Something stand-out but smart can only be a good thing on your first day.

DON'T...

• Go all-out with your best Friday-night face. You'll get to know the lay of the land within a couple of weeks. It's best to start in a safe makeup place and work up from there.
• Forget you've got it on and eat a burrito for lunch. An oily lipstick print on your chin in your afternoon meetings might undo all your hard work.

BIG MEETING/
PRESENTATION

Listen, makeup power players do exist. We've seen it backstage, we've seen it IRL, lord knows we've seen it in the 1980s. If you want to feel confident and appear impressive, try one of the following...

POWER BROW

This means defined from the arch to the end, and natural at the front. Your brows are expressive. Keeping them strong and groomed will let them do some of the talking.

BOLD LIP

If you have 12 people in one conference room, and one of them is wearing Ruby Woo to a fault, who is going to stand out? Use this knowledge to your advantage.

CONTOUR

A subtle contour will enhance your cheekbones, set your makeup off right and make you feel pulled together. Use a cream contour stick under the cheek bones and blend to add a soft structure.

AS MUCH AS PEOPLE TALK ABOUT BEAUTY
ADVICE FOR EVERY OCCASION, NO ONE
CONCENTRATES ON THE UNDOINGS.
THE THINGS THAT CAN PLAY HAVOC
WITH YOUR DAY, YOUR LIFE, YOUR FACE.
YOU CAN BE PREPARED FOR EVERY DAY,
THIS SECTION MIGHT BE THE MOST USEFUL YET.
WE'RE PUTTING THE REAL IN REAL LIFE.

THE

DISRUP

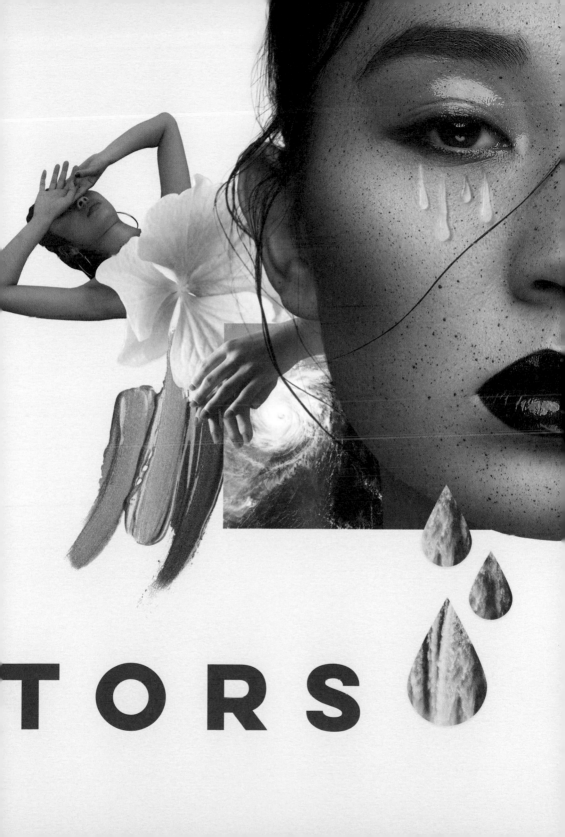

PERIODS

HI THERE HORMONES.

IT'S KIND OF
YOU TO WANT TO DROP IN ONCE A MONTH,
AND YES WE NEED YOU,
BUT WE DON'T LIKE YOU.

IF YOU COULD JUST TRY TO KEEP THINGS
A BIT LESS PROBLEMATIC NEXT TIME YOU
VISIT THAT WOULD BE GREAT, THANKS.

Want to know why periods are associated with spots? It's the oestrogen and progesterone hormone battle. Knowledge is power, if you understand why your face is freaking out, you can take steps to make it better.

WEEK BEFORE YOUR PERIOD

Progesterone and testosterone are peaking around now, and this is where most of your skin woes come from. Progesterone actually makes your skin inflamed and your sebaceous glands produce more oil, which then gets trapped under your inflamed (therefore tighter) pores. Dead skin cells and bacteria get involved and then, wham, a spot is born.

WHAT TO DO

Try not to cover your spots if you can help it (if you need to cover them, page 15 tells you how). Help your skin cells turnover and your pores clear with an acid toner like Caudalie Vinopure Clear Skin Purifying Toner. Sounds scary – really isn't. But only use it twice a week if you've never used one before.

WEEK OF YOUR PERIOD

As soon as you start bleeding your skin should start improving. Your body is now producing oestrogen, which counteracts the progesterone and kind of dries your skin out. You'll probably feel grim, but at least your skin is about to enter healing mode.

WHAT TO DO

Treat every day like it's Skincare Sunday (i.e. indulge your skin to the max), but include chocolate and a hot water bottle, too. Your skin will benefit, your mood will benefit, your mouth will benefit – as will your stomach.

WEEK AFTER YOUR PERIOD

Your body is getting ready to ovulate again, so your oestrogen levels are rising and progesterone dropping. This is about where your skin is its clearest so make the most of it. Go out? Go on a date? At the very least take some selfies.

WHAT TO DO

Properly hydrate your skin, cos the oestrogen is drying it out. A mask will do it, as will drinking lots of water or, if we're getting serious, hyaluronic acid serum.

SOPHIE LOVES: SkinCeuticals Hydrating B5.

LISA LOVES: Elemis Hydra-Boost Serum.

> *S.B.* I have endometriosis, so I have horrendous periods that can last up to twelve days. My main focus is just carrying on with life and getting through the pain, but doing my makeup or a proper skincare session does always make me feel better, as do very hot baths and watching Sex & The City episodes back to back. Could I be any more clichéd?

ALLERGIES

NO ONE WILL EVER UNDERSTAND
THAT DISRUPTIVE IRRITATION OF ITCHY,
STREAMING EYES UNTIL THEY'VE EXPERIENCED
THEM.

IF YOU CARRY AN EMERGENCY
SUPPLY OF PIRITON AT ALL TIMES,
YOU WILL APPRECIATE THE NEED
FOR THE NEXT COUPLE OF PAGES.

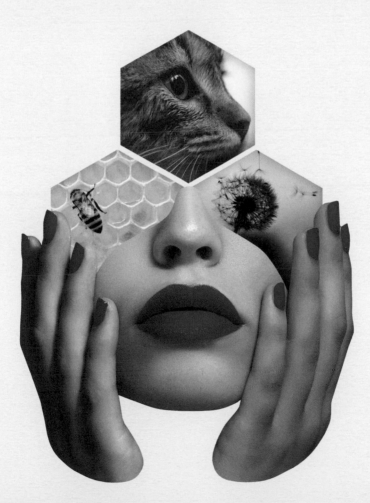

> *S.B.* My biggest fear in life was to fall in love with someone who was allergic to cats. Thank god that didn't happen.

> *L.P.D.* I have horrendous hay fever, it's the most annoying thing. You feel like you've got a head cold for months. I will always itch off my concealer, I cry my mascara off all summer and what makes it worse is pollen can get stuck behind my contact lenses. So yeah. I look great in summer.

Allergies, be they from pets, dust, hay fever, nuts, false nails, are an absolute pain in the beauty behind. You cannot plan when you will cross paths with a hairy dachshund or accidentally eat crustaceans (that might result in A&E, we are not suggesting makeup can help with that), but if you are faced with an allergic reaction, here is how to minimize the makeup fallout.

COMMON SYMPTOMS

SNEEZING AND AN ITCHY, RUNNY OR BLOCKED NOSE

Paw paw cream around the base of your nose acts as a pollen barrier and keeps the area hydrated so it doesn't crack. Counteract the redness using a yellow-toned creamy concealer that won't dry out, and press in with clean fingers.

ITCHY, RED, WATERING EYES

Always carry eye drops. Put cucumber in the fridge to take down swollen eyes in the morning, and/or use an eye mask that you keep in the freezer. Lisa swears by these over summer.

Actually avoid mascara – if you rub it into your eyes it can make it worse in the short and the long term. Just do a stronger brow to give focus to your eye area. Get your lashes tinted before hay fever season, so you can go makeup-free as much as possible.

A RAISED, ITCHY, RED RASH OR HIVES

Try Sudocrem – it's a beauty insider's must-have. It contains zinc to counteract the inflammation, and since it's formulated for babies, it's good for highly sensitive skin. Use at night rather than the day.

If you need to leave the house, try mineral makeup. Again, the natural zinc helps with inflammation and the finely milled powder gives decent coverage whilst letting your skin breathe.

SWOLLEN LIPS

Go with it. People pay good money for that. Joking, obviously. Go to the doctors – any kind of swelling might get worse before it gets better, so better to be safe than sorry.

FYI: Some people are actually allergic to makeup. If that is you, we are sorry from the bottom of our hearts, and we hope that this book has at least been entertaining if not practical.

CRYING

IF YOU NEED TO READ THIS CHAPTER
WE HOPE YOU'RE OK. BUT MAYBE YOU'RE
CRYING WITH LAUGHTER. OR MAYBE
YOU JUST WATCHED MARLEY AND ME
IN AN AIRPLANE WITH RED WINE – THE MOST
TEAR-INDUCING COMBINATION EVER. EITHER WAY,
WE'RE HERE TO HELP.

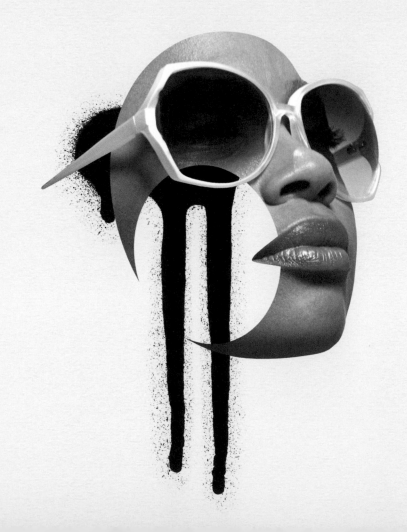

UGLY CRYING

Tears are not just sat there waiting to happen. When you cry the fluid has to come from somewhere, and that way is through the blood vessels around your eyes so they dilate and become more prominent. Hence the redness and puffiness.

Extra blood rushes into your face and nose when you cry, making it hot and red. Sometimes your nose inflames and gets blocked entirely.

Your breathing becomes irregular and when you hold your breath for any reason you slow the blood flow to your lungs, so again, vessels dilate and you go red. And puffy. Yey.

Crying triggers the tearing reflex and muscle scrunching, so you contort your face to push tears up and out of your tear ducts. Ugly but true.

HOW TO COMBAT CRYING FACE

Try and stand outside or splash your face with water to cool down and allow the colour to return to normal. In fact, splashing with water might be the best thing, because then you can redo your makeup instead of trying to salvage it. Dead give away.

Take some really deep breaths to decompress and calm your whole body. Your colour and emotional demeanour will (hopefully) soon return to normal.

Nude – not white – eyeliner in the waterline will take down the appearance of redness and brighten your eyes without looking too obvious.

Jet-black mascara is going to redefine your eyes, separate your lashes after the tears might have clumped them together (may be worth touching your lashes onto dry tissue to soak up the excess tears first), and put you back together again.

Gold eyeshadow (or something with a subtle sheen) will open your eyes up, and the warmth will enhance your eye colour, rather than the redness in the whites of the eyes.

So next time you feel you're about to emotionally overflow, take a time-out to build and collect your anti-crying makeup kit. By the time you're done you might have distracted yourself enough that the tears don't come in the first place. Win win.

THE BACKCHAT BEAUTY ANTI-CRYING KIT:

Nude liner	NYX Professional Makeup Wonder Pencil.
Cry-proof mascara	Benefit BADgal BANG!
Gold shadow	Charlotte Tilbury Luxury Palette The Golden Goddess.
Calming spray	Neal's Yard Remedies White Tea Facial Mist.

The good news is, ugly crying has an evolutionary purpose for humans. It makes you more likely to receive sympathy from people around you. Hugs save lives.

HANG-OVERS

A FEW TOO MANY DRINKS LAST NIGHT
EQUALS NOT THE BEST YOU IN THE MORNING.
DON'T PANIC, YOU CAN FIX THAT.
ALSO APPLIES TO RECOVERY FROM FLU, LACK
OF SLEEP AND BINGE-WATCHING BOX SETS.

L.P.D. My worst hangover was at uni, I drunk a bottle
of red wine (I hate wine), but it was cheap (I was at uni).
I threw up the bottle of wine – it was luminous pink
on the way out – and I fell asleep in my student shower
which was communal.
I was woken the next day by a concerned student
(non-drinker, hard-worker) who needed to check
I was still breathing before he got in the shower.
I've never drunk wine since.

S.B. The only thing worse than a severe hangover
is trying to conceal it from your colleagues.
My skin goes grey and makeup just sort of sits on
top of it like a hangover beacon, rather than the gentle
enhancing job it does every other day. This is because
of the dehydration. So my tips start the night before.

SKINCARE

Your skin is parched. This may not always be possible (which
is why we have trained our husbands to do it for us if necessary),
but take your makeup off before sleep. Your skin needs to breathe
and repair, which it concentrates on overnight. Leaving a layer
of, essentially, dirt on the skin isn't going to let that happen.

Then add a mask.

No one is going to do that.

OK, at least a night cream.

BASE

Wear a liquid highlighter under your foundation. It gives the
illusion of a dewy glow, i.e. like you've had eight hours sleep.

Apply concealer all the way around the eyes, under your lashes
and on the lids. When dehydrated, this area is much darker.

Stay away from matte foundation, your skin will already be looking a little flat, stick to a dewy liquid foundation or a tinted moisturizer.

EYES

Use a nude liner in the waterline – not white, it makes eyes look smaller – to counteract redness and make you look more awake.

Try a blue mascara, rather than black – it brightens the whites of your eyes.

CHEEKS

Put colour back in your face. A touch of coral/orange cream blusher gives a naturally dewy finish and is an easy brightening cheat that suits most skin tones.

LIPS

Avoid colour, you don't want to draw too much attention to your face, but go for a tinted balm that will make them look hydrated and healthy.

> If you've been drinking red wine, embrace the stain, you can put a clear balm over the top.

> Unless you're me, then don't drink the red wine in the first place.

> My worst hangover, by the way, was my second day at ELLE. My new team had taken me out for welcome drinks the night before, and I couldn't be publicly hungover this early into the job. Top tip: Always find out where the disabled toilets are on your first day – the privacy will be invaluable on your second day, when you discover an intolerance to team mojitos, but you need to maintain professionalism and respect... Blusher and a fake smile also helps.

RAIN

WEATHER IN GENERAL CAN DISRUPT
OUR BEST-LAID BEAUTY PLANS,
BUT GOD DAMN YOU RAIN, YOU ARE
THE ABSOLUTE WORST. SHORT OF CARRYING
A PLASTIC DOTTY RAIN CAP LIKE
LISA'S NAN DORIS (GENIUS, WE SHOULD BRING
THOSE BACK) IN CASE OF A DOWNPOUR,
THERE ARE PREVENTATIVE STEPS YOU
CAN TAKE TO AVOID A BEAUTY CATASTROPHE,
AND THEN QUICK TRICKS TO GET
YOUR LOOK BACK ON TRACK.

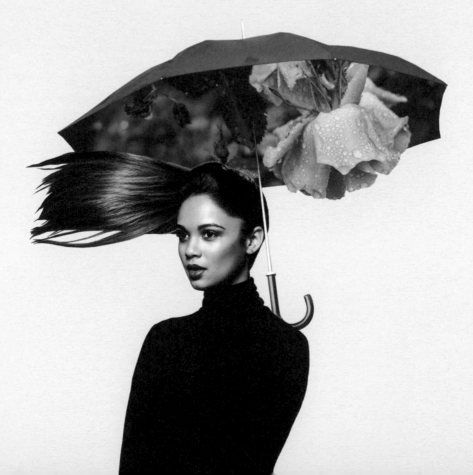

It's easy to protect your makeup in the rain, just look down, so what we really need to solve here is the hair situation.

The only problem really is if you've spent ages getting your texture right without checking the weather app or looking out the window. The rain will undo all the work. If your hair is styled in an updo, it shouldn't really matter too much.

If you tong your texture in (like us), twist your finished hair into a bun. That way if it rains, leave it, let it dry and when you let it out it should have retained most of the wave.

Braids. The bonus hairstyle with benefits. That being, braids look great, but then when you let them dry in and take them out they look even better. Try two low plaits at the back, twist them together at the nape of your neck for a bohemian style. They'll look great with or without rain, and be weatherproof, too.

> *S.B.* I went for a blowdry in New York during Fashionweek, and it started raining when I was on my way to a show. Luckily I'd been to Glossier earlier, so I emptied my bag and put the whole thing on my head. It wasn't the chicest, but at least I was somewhere I didn't know anyone. That is until someone DMs me to say they'd passed me in Tribecca with a bag on my head. Joy!

It's raining. You have options here...

EMBRACE THE RAIN

Imagine a scenario where you've spent half an hour tonging your hair and you're on your way somewhere nice. You have no umbrella, what do you do?

> *L.P.D.* I take my hair out and slick it back with my hands, then gather into a ponytail and add red lipstick like it's a Spanish thing. I make the wetness central to the look. The only problem is having to keep going and re-wetting it in the toilet all day. Maybe I embrace it a bit too much.

CONTROL THE FRIZZ

OK, so it's wet, it's not what you were going for but it will dry! Only it will dry wrong if you have that kind of hair. Unless you do this, that is.

> My hair is prone to frizziness, but I love a natural finish too. When my hair gets unexpectedly ruined by the rain, I put it into a middle parting, then take small sections and twist them tightly round my fingers, then gather the twists into a loose pony. When they're dry I take it out, shake through with my fingers and probably have better hair than I did when I left the house in the first place.

BE RESOURCEFUL WITH THE DRYING OPTIONS

The hand dryers in the public loos are basically the same as your hairdryer but a different shape. You will need to leave your dignity in the cubicle, get your head under the air and put a pile of paper towels next to you to give the people who need to actually dry their hands. Whilst drying, rake the roots taut with your fingers for extra shine, and scrunch the ends for a tousled finish. Embarrassing, maybe. Effective, definitely.

As there are mini makeup products, there are mini hair products that can save you in rainy situations. A serum or texture spray will finish off your look to make it look like this was the style you were going for all along. Us 1, rain nil.

HEART-BREAK

SH*T HAPPENS. YOU HAVE TWO OPTIONS.
GET IN BED AND CRY UNTIL YOUR MASCARA
STAINS YOUR PILLOW. OR, PUT ON
A HAPPY FACE, LITERALLY. HERE'S HOW.

·This isn't us telling you to cheer up, love (which FYI is exactly the wrong thing to say to anyone, ever).

It's us reminding you to never forget how good you can feel. You know how buying an amazing new outfit makes you want to go out in it? You need the makeup equivalent of that.

COLOUR

There is actual psychological reasoning about colour, it's called Chromotherapy, so basically, what we're telling you is we're scientists now (see page 50).

SKIN

Treat yo'self. Sheet masks are the most indulgent pick-me-up in packet form. You need some 'me-time', and 15 minutes should just about do it (with better skin as a bonus).

FACE

Bronzer is your best friend. Think of it like this; everyone feels their best in summer with a bit of colour, so whether it's real or fake, a warm glow will give you that emotional boost.

EYES

The windows to your soul, and the biggest giveaway to your broken heart, so dress them up in the most flamboyant curtains possible. Be that a royal blue mascara, a jade green liner or a purple smoky eye.

> *L.P.D.* As a makeup artist I relate to the importance of colour. Green is one of my go-to shades, and according to chromotherapy it supports harmony and love. So that works.

LIPS

The best place to go bright. It gives a very simple confidence boost, lights your whole face, makes you look groomed and generally like you have your sh*t together. Nervous? Start with a universally flattering coral and pat it on using your finger. Work up from there.

> *S.B.* Red lipstick is my metaphorical medicine. If I'm tired, sad, nervous or rolling on the ground in emotional agony, I literally will wear nothing else, just to test its super powers.

VITAL: Don't give up on yourself. Whatever the reason for your heartbreak, treat every day like you're going to bump into your ex – i.e. look great, feel better, and remember, this is for you and no one else.

> When you're going through hard times, and every day can bring potential heartbreak, you learn to love longwear. I am heavily reliant on lipstick, because I can't physically cry it off.

> Once, when I was a teenager, I cried so much that all my glitter eye makeup went into my eyes and got stuck behind my contacts and I had to get medical assistance. Which was frankly more upsetting than the thing that made me cry in the first place.

RUSH HOUR

NO MATTER HOW MUCH TIME YOU'VE SPENT
GETTING READY IN THE MORNING,
YOU CANNOT ACCOUNT FOR THE DREADED
RUSH HOUR. WILL YOUR FACE BE JAMMED IN
SOMEONE'S ARMPIT? WILL YOU BE
DOING YOUR MAKEUP IN THE PASSENGER SEAT?
WILL THE AIR CON BE BROKEN?
OR WORSE, WILL THE HEATING BE ON?

S.B. I know I've come undone when it gets to the point where sweat is trickling down my back. No one can maintain any beauty decorum when their back is wet.

L.P.D. If you are lucky enough to live in London and ever get the Central Line, DO NOT touch ANYTHING. Once, I was on my way out – I'd made a big effort with my hair and makeup, and noticed everyone was staring at me. I thought, 'Oh I must really look nice. How nice'. I got my phone out to do an Instastory when I got off, and my entire face was covered in black marks. Jet black, from touching my face after touching the pole. Now, forget about how I looked. There's a thing called girl code, girls. If you see someone compromised like that on the tube, tell them.

What if they thought it was part of your look?

Come on now, I looked like an American footballer. I looked like I was going into battle. No.

COMBAT THE COMMUTE

The things you need to keep your beauty cool on the move...

☐ A FAN

The paper kind, not the 'you're the greatest, you can get through this' kind.

☐ COOLING MIST OR BALM

To apply to your face (or inside your wrists or back of your neck – great tip for quicker cooling). Try La Roche Posay Thermal Spring Water Face Mist, Mario Badescu Facial Spray with Aloe Herbs and Rosewater or Milk Makeup Cooling Water.

☐ SETTING SPRAY

This will help keep your makeup on through the sweating, but also stop it transferring onto the shoulder shoved in your face. We like Urban Decay All Nighter and MAC Prep + Prime Fix +.

☐ HALO BRAID

Keep your hair off your forehead with this style. This allows you to sweat freely without worrying about frizzing, but also diminishes sweating because your neck will be cooler, too.

☐ COOLING EYE MAKEUP CRAYONS

A new revelation for people like Sophie, who do their makeup on the train.

> *S.B.* I do my make up on the move wherever possible, and I use Dior cooling eye stick. It's like having your eyelids licked by a unicorn. And it looks amazing and blends perfectly. And it's waterproof so it stays there. Lisa thought I was mad, I made her try it, and she agrees about the unicorn thing.

☐ HAND SANITIZER

You have to assume that whoever sat in that seat before you did not have the same hygiene standards as you. Best to sanitize and be safe before you touch your face. Also, check for black marks.

☐ MINIS

Most brands are now doing minis. Uber-portable makeup is your rush hour best friend – whether you do your whole face on your way in with it, or you need easy access to reapply or touch up whatever has suffered during your journey. This is how to beat rush hour beautifully.

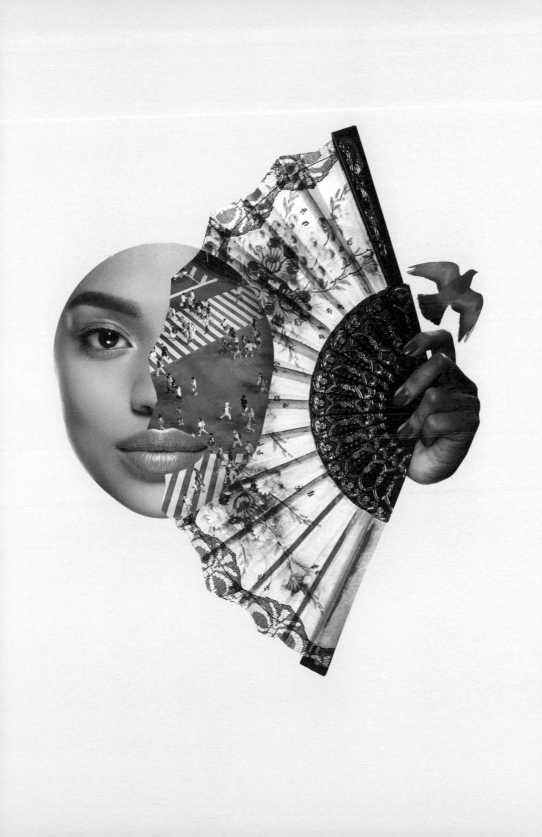

OUR FAVOURITE MINIS:

- Benefit BADgal BANG!
- Mac Mini Lipsticks
- BECCA Backlight Primer
- Hourglass Ambient Light Mini

If you work at a desk, have emergency makeup in your drawers. That way you don't have to carry heavy makeup in your bag and therefore take up more space on the train. You will more than likely need to top up what you've sweated off when you get to work anyway.

BAD EYESIGHT

BAD EYESIGHT OR GOOD OPPORTUNITY TO WEAR AMAZING GLASSES? YOU DECIDE, BUT FOR THE RECORD, WE ARE SAYING THE LATTER. WE BOTH WEAR PRESCRIPTION GLASSES, AND CONTACT LENSES WHEN WE WANT A CHANGE. OUR MAKEUP ALSO NEEDS SOME AMENDING IN THAT CASE. HERE'S HOW.

GLASSES WEARERS

Get a magnifying mirror – because you can't apply your makeup with your glasses on. One for the bathroom, and a hand-held one for your makeup bag. Game changer.

If you're blessed with great lashes, curl them, otherwise they'll touch the glass, smudge the lenses and imprint mascara where you don't want it.

Counteract the shadow or discolouration caused by frames by concealing under the eye with a product one shade lighter than your complexion. This will brighten your eyes instantly.

If you're a liner lover, match your frame size to your liner. This means if you wear a heavy dark frame, you should wear a thicker line to make the eye stand out. Otherwise your glasses can overpower your face. If it's a thinner frame, make the liner finer and softer.

Define your brows. You won't want them to get lost behind your frames. This makes the biggest difference when you're wearing glasses.

S.B. I always look better in my glasses if I do a simple one-tone smoke with kohl in the waterline. It's just about extra definition of my eyes so they don't get lost behind the glasses.

L.P.D. I always highlight the inner corner of my eye to add an extra brightness behind the lenses.

CONTACT LENS WEARERS

Essentially contact lens makeup is the same as any makeup, except you need to think a little more about makeup. Don't worry, it's not a big deal, you just need a little more care, and yes, you can still wear glitter.

First thing first. Put your lenses in a decent amount of time before you start your makeup, let them settle in and then begin.

If you can avoid makeup that touches the lenses – like kohl in the waterline – do that. But if it's key to your look, don't worry too much. The worst that can happen is your lenses get dirty and can irritate. In which case you need to clean or change them. Which is tricky to do without messing up your makeup.

Don't wiggle your mascara wand right into the root. You can still get excellent definition by applying from mid-lengths to the tips.

On that note, always replace your mascara every three months, no matter the brand. This goes for everyone, but particularly lens wearers. Old mascaras are prone to flaking into the eye and can cause infection.

Take your lenses out before you remove your makeup, because you need to rub your eyes and you'll just irritate them otherwise.

Oh, and always wash your hands before you touch your eyes. But you knew that anyway.

> I love wearing glasses. Except when you go into a bar in winter and you fog up for a good ten minutes before you regain composure. That is the exact opposite of cool.

THE O
OF-OF

EVERYTHING YOU NEED FOR A
DAY OFF AT HOME, TO A FULL-ON HOLIDAY.
ALL OUR TRAVEL, PACKING AND SUN-SAVING
BEAUTY TIPS FOR STAYCATIONING OR
VACATIONING ARE HERE. ENJOY YOUR TRIP!
SEND US A POSTCARD NEXT TIME…

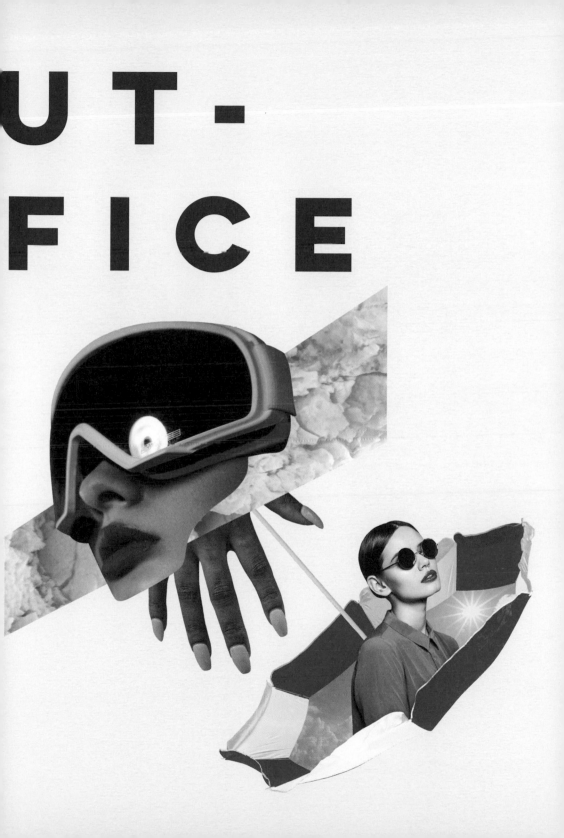

TOP TRAVEL PRODUCTS

LISA

DESTINATION: IBIZA

Ibiza is one of my favourite places in the universe. I'm not talking hardcore rave Ibiza, I'm talking, lively beach club parties where you stand out if you're NOT head to toe in glitter. This is my five-day edit of everything I take to the White Isle.

- ☐ SPF 50 for body – Ultrasun Sports Spray.
- ☐ SPF 50 for face – La Roche Posay Anthelios XL Ultra Light Tinted Fluid.
- ☐ SPF 30 lip balm – Fresh Sugar Sport Treatment.
- ☐ Cleanser – Elemis Pro-Collagen Cleansing Balm (takes off everything – even glitter).
- ☐ Moisturizer (decanted if only staying a few days; a full pot if longer) – Hada Labo Tokyo Skin Plumping Gel Cream.
- ☐ Body moisturizer (decanted) – Brazilian Bum Bum Cream.
- ☐ Liquid bronzer – TIME BOMB Cosmetics Holiday In a Bottle.
- ☐ Concealer – NARS Radiant Creamy Concealer.
- ☐ Brow gel – Benefit Gimme Brow+.
- ☐ Cream blush and lip combo – Charlotte Tilbury Beach Stick in Las Salinas (also an amazing beach in Ibiza).
- ☐ Glitter and glue – Eco Glitter and The Gypsy Shrine.
- ☐ Orange eyeliner – MAC Chromagraphic Pencil in Genuine Orange.
- ☐ Eyeshadow palette – Pat McGrath Mothership II Sublime Palette.
- ☐ Mascara – Benefit BADgal BANG!
- ☐ Hat – essential to protect your face.
- ☐ Hair tong – GHD Classic Curve.
- ☐ Dry shampoo – Living Proof Perfect Hair Day.

SOPHIE

DESTINATION: NEW YORK

I go to NYC twice a year minimum, so I've got my packing down. I use multi-tasking products, so I don't have to pack heavy, I'm more drawn to bright colour when I'm away, but mostly I make sure I've ticked off every skin eventuality in mini saviour form.

- ☐ SPF 50 – Obagi Medical Sun Shield Tint.
- ☐ Perfume – Ex Nihilo Fleur Narcotique.
- ☐ Rehydration sachets.
- ☐ Cleanser – mini Cetaphil cleanser.
- ☐ Muslin cloth.
- ☐ Serums – SkinCeuticals Hydrating B5 and CE Ferulic.
- ☐ Moisturizer – Sisley mini.
- ☐ Mini Sudocrem.
- ☐ La Roche Posay Effaclar IA.
- ☐ Texture spray – Mini Sam McKnight Cool Girl Barely There Texture Mist.
- ☐ Hairspray – Mini L'Oreal Elnett Hairspray.
- ☐ Wrinkle releaser – Downy Wrinkle Releaser (from USA).
- ☐ Hair styler – GHD Curve Classic Wave Wand with US plug.
- ☐ Lip crayons – Crayola Lip Crayon in Red and Bronze.
- ☐ Mascara – YSL Mascara in Blue.
- ☐ Lipstick – Laura Mercier Velour Exteme Matte Lip in Stylin.
- ☐ Lips and eyes – Clarins 4-colour Pen for Eyes and Lips.
- ☐ Brow-styling – Benefit Brow Contour Pro.

PRE-HOLIDAY PREP

YOU'VE PLANNED, YOU'VE PACKED
(OR YOU'VE PLANNED TO PACK),
AND NOW IT'S TIME TO PREP.
PRE-HOLIDAY TENDS TO BE LAST MINUTE
BUT THESE ARE THE THINGS WE SUGGEST YOU
TRY TO FIT IN IF YOU CAN.

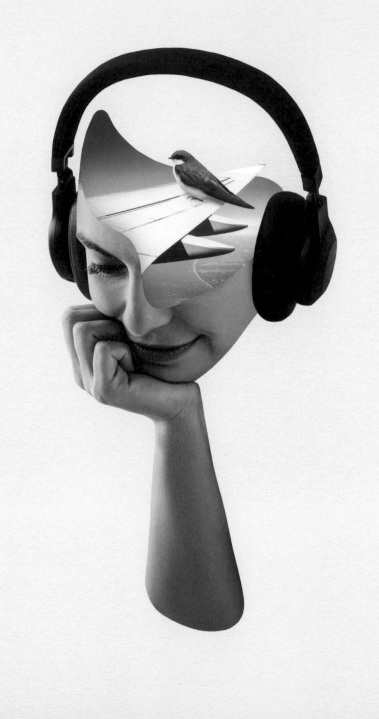

☐ GET A SPRAY TAN

Why? No one wants to be the palest person in the place (plus it adds a beautiful healthy ironically post-holiday glow to your skin).

☐ GO FOR GEL NAILS

Why? They will last at least a two-week holiday without having to worry.

☐ HAVE A PROPER PEDI

Why? We're talking the heel-shaving, soft-skin, foot facial. Your holiday wardrobe will always look better with a pedicure.

☐ HAIR: ROOT TOUCH UP AND TRIM

Why? We live in the Instagram age. Photos will more than likely help you capture your memories. Visible roots and split ends are not compatible with the 'gram.

☐ WAXING

Why? Because you're going to be wearing less than normal, so you will want no stragglers on show, or to waste time shaving when you could be drinking sangrias.

☐ LASH EXTENSIONS

Why? Not an essential, but you'll wake up feeling made up, so you can get straight out onto the beach. (Once you've SPFed.)

IN-FLIGHT PACKING LIST:

- ☐ Sheet mask.
- ☐ Aromatherapy roller for pulse points.
- ☐ Mini packet eye makeup remover wipes.
- ☐ Phone charger and worldwide adapter.
- ☐ Your fave foundation.
- ☐ Your fave moisturizer.
- ☐ Concealer.
- ☐ Retractable foundation brush or Beautyblender.
- ☐ Hydration spray.
- ☐ Immune-boosting vitamins (Airbourne or Berocca).
- ☐ Chewing gum or mints.
- ☐ Paracetamol.
- ☐ Ear plugs.
- ☐ Lip balm with SPF.

FOR AN HOUR BEFORE YOU LAND

- ☐ Lip and cheek tint.
- ☐ Mini mascara (try NARS Climax Mascara).
- ☐ Hand mirror.
- ☐ Brow gel (try Benefit 24 Hour Brow Setter).
- ☐ Toothbrush and mini toothpaste.
- ☐ Powder foundation and foundation brush (try bareMinerals Original Foundation SPF 15).

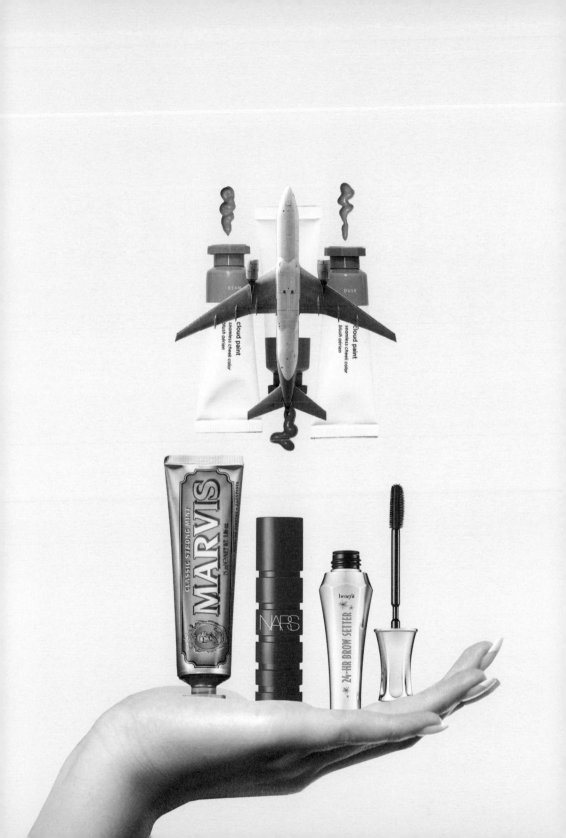

IN THE HEAT

WHETHER YOU'RE CHASING THE SUN
OR BASKING IN YOUR BACK GARDEN,
ALL SIGNS POINT TO THE FACT YOU
WANT SERIOUS HEAT ON YOUR SKIN.
CLOTHES, NO PROBLEM (MINIMAL),
MAKEUP AND HAIR, HOWEVER, CAN
BE TRICKIER. HERE'S OUR GUIDE
TO STYLING OUT THE SUNSHINE.

SKIN

Let's get this out the way because you know we're going to find out where you live and beat you with your washbag otherwise. ALWAYS USE SPF – turn to page 145.

Can we just talk about Freckles, please?

> *S.B.* I get a cute smattering of freckles across my nose as soon as my face sees the sun, I bloody love them. Makes me feel about ten years younger, too.

> *L.P.D.* I am obsessed with freckles, I even draw them in sometimes. If you have them, embrace them! Please don't cover them up.

> So long as they are well protected with SPF 50, you're lucky if you have them!

Rosehip oil is a great 'dry' oil, so the perfect nourishing product to add to your routine – it'll counter any dehydration, and won't feel or look greasy on the skin. So good for dry or humid heat. Best to apply when your skin is slightly damp after cleansing to trap extra moisture in the skin.

WE LOVE: Trilogy Rosehip Oil Light Blend and The Ordinary 100% Organic Cold-Pressed Rosehip Seed Oil.

If you tend to feel clogged by SPF or sweat, try a gentle enzyme mask at the end of the day. Don't go for harsh acids, just natural fruit enzymes that will gently dissolve the top layer of dead skin and dirt so your pores are free! Sophie uses Elemis Papaya Enzyme Peel every day whilst away.

Mattifying. Well, not completely, because flat matte skin isn't the thing. Embrace the glow! But if it gets too much, try this:

• An oil control moisturizer or primer where you get shiny.
• Paula's Choice Shine Stopper.
• The Body Shop Seaweed Oil-Control Gel Cream.

If you're out and about and need to take the shine down, a mineral blotting powder is great (has a low level natural SPF and lets your skin breathe), but we also heard a rumour that cigarette Rizla papers are the absolute best blotting tool there is. Amazingly cheap, conveniently tiny. Do not smoke. Ever.

WE LOVE: bareMinerals Invisible Light Translucent Powder Duo – absorbs oil and gives a fresh not flat finish.

MAKEUP

The vitamin D does wonders for your complexion, so embrace it. Swap your foundation for a tinted moisturizer, or thin out your foundation by mixing it with a touch of moisturizer before you apply.

A touch of safe tanning from the sun will look even better with bright colours on your eyes and lips. But keep makeup minimal – a full face looks out of place on the beach, plus anything that stops you being able to run into the sea should stay at home!

> *L.P.D.* I love blue mascara every day, but it looks incredible when the sun hits it, especially if it's the only makeup on your face.

> *S.B.* I rarely go a summer's day without bright coral lipstick and nothing else. Warms up my whole face and makes me happy when I look at it.

That would also actually look great on your cheeks. You can do the matchy matchy multi-tasking thing in summer.

Lips can sometimes suffer in the heat. Use an SPF balm to help protect the moisture in your lips, and also give a little healthy sheen. It'll mean any lip colour you follow it with will also look better.

HAIR

If you're at the beach you have the world's best hair-styling product right in front of you. In abundance. Get in the sea, let your hair down and dry it naturally in the sun for the most amazing natural texture. You can twist small sections as it dries for a little more control.

When you go out and want it a little more 'finished', use the sea texture as a base, then take small random sections from the top and curl with heat protection spray and tongs for a more defined look.

Braids keep your hair off your face and neck, keep your texture under control and can stay in for days. Pick a flower and tuck it behind your ear for extra holiday vibes.

CHILL OUT

GONE SKIING? GONE TO RUSSIA?
GONE TO LONDON ON BANK HOLIDAY?
HERE'S HOW TO DEAL WITH
YOUR FACE IN THE COLD.

L.P.D. I've never been skiing, but I've been to Chamonix when it was fully snowing. It was amaaazing.

S.B. Why weren't you skiing?

Didn't fancy it.

SKIN

The good news is, everyone officially looks cute in the cold. Something about being bundled up in layers of knitwear, with rosy cheeks and a pink tip of the nose. But just as the heat can be hard on your skin, so can the cold.

Again. SPF. We can't say it enough, all year round, but if you're skiing? Well that's equivalent to being naked on a sailing boat in high summer. The snow acts as a reflector, intensifying the UVA and UVB rays onto your skin, hence the famous goggle masks. Protect yourself before you wreck yourself (see page 145).

Wind is abrasive, beating it is all about protecting your moisture barrier. That is your natural protective layer that keeps the bad stuff (irritants and bacteria) out and the good stuff (moisture) in. Wind can dry out the outer layers of your skin, almost like a harsh natural exfoliation – but not in a good way.

There are products that repair or even mimic your moisture barrier, now is the time to add them in.

SOPHIE LOVES: Avene Skin Recovery Cream.
LISA LOVES: Egyptian Magic All Purpose Cream.

Afterburn. You might not see it like sunburn, but if your skin has red patches, is sensitive, itchy or dry, you can soothe it just as you would with aftersun. Natural aloe vera is best, but in the absence of an aloe plant in the middle of a sub-zero ski resort, use organic natural paw paw cream – specifically designed for minor cuts, scratches and abrasions.

Lips suffer first in cold weather; moisture is easily lost here so they get dry and chapped. A good barrier function lip balm is key to stop moisture getting out.

SOPHIE LOVES: Aquaphor Lip Repair.
LISA LOVES: Ultrasun Lip Protection SPF 30.

Your hands will need some extra care in the cold. Something multi-tasking like Neutrogena Norwegian Formula Concentrated Handcream will help nourish the skin and nails, whilst protecting the skin barrier even in the harshest conditions. Like Sophie's air-conditioned office.

TIP: Apply to your feet at night, wear socks and be prepared to wake up with baby soft feet.

HAIR

Cold is one thing, wind is another, together it's quite a beauty-wrecking combo.

> *S.B.* I've been caught in a New York snow blizzard before. My hair actually froze and snapped. I keep it all under a hat these days.

You'll want to keep your hair in place to avoid being whipped round the face, or arriving looking bedraggled and totally come-undone. Of course you can just slick it back and pin any straggling bits in place. Or you could try a wind-proof style.

Try gathering hair into a low or side ponytail, pull out the front section, twist round your finger then pin back into the ponytail. Any bits the wind wisps up will add to the romance of the look.

Leave-in conditioner is a winter winner; it's more nourishing than your normal conditioner because it doesn't get washed out, and since cold, dry air sucks moisture from your hair, you'll appreciate it. Similarly, a hair mask once a week is going to keep it shiny and healthy.

HOW TO DEAL WITH HAT HAIR

Keep your ears warm, make it work with your hair. Either establish a flat-roots style (curl the ends only and let the hat flatten the top), or pull hair into two fishtail braids that will look great with or without a woolly hat. Basically you need to go low with your styling, anything that starts at the nape of the neck is most compatible with hats. Low pony, loose low bun or knot, side braid, anything.

MAKEUP

If you're prone to redness anyway, the cold might make it worse. Use a YSL peach-toned colour corrector under your foundation; it'll give a glow to your skin even if you don't have any redness.

It's really nice to add a tiny bit of sheer highlighter to the apples of your cheeks to make your skin a little bit glassy. It works well with the natural high colour you'll have from the cold.

Go for lip balm over lip gloss to avoid your hair sticking to it. In fact, a tinted balm is the nicest and most helpful. Matte colour will make your dry lips even drier, satin might highlight any cracks or flaky skin and gloss we've already covered. Those pH colour-changing balms are a nice option for a perfect bespoke finish.

LISA LOVES: Winky Lux Jelly pH Lip Balm.
SOPHIE LOVES: Dior Addict Lip Glow.

Waterproof coloured liner is a good option in the cold. Eyes tend to water when you're cold, so smoke or mascara-heavy makeup is a bit trickier. If you concentrate on the top lid, above the lashes and use a good longwear formula, you'll be fine. Colour adds some skin-perking interest.

LISA LOVES: Urban Decay 24/7 Glide-On Eye Pencil.
SOPHIE LOVES: Dior Diorshow On Stage Liner.

SPF

JUST DO IT.
HERE ARE THE BASICS.

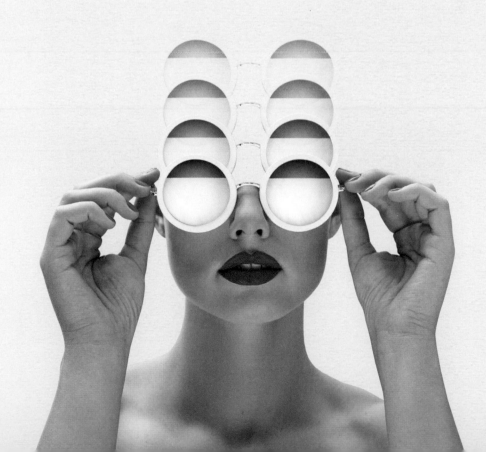

UVA V.S. UVB

Stands for long-wave Ultra Violet A and short-wave Ultra
Violet B. Remember it this way – UVA is for ageing. UVB is
for burning.

The A rays penetrate into the deeper layers of your skin, causing
wrinkles and ageing.

The B rays burn the more superficial layers, and can cause cancer.

Up to 20% of harmful rays can penetrate the skin, even on a
cloudy day. Always use a broad-spectrum sunscreen that covers
both.

THE RULES

1. UVA is equally intense in winter, even on cloudy days, so
always use SPF.

2. Use at least SPF 30, which blocks 97% of the sun's UVB rays.

3. Apply half an hour before sun exposure.

4. Use more than you think you need:
• Half a teaspoon on your face alone.
• Two teaspoons for head, arms and neck (clothed).
• Two tablespoons if covering entire body (in swimsuit).

5. Reapply every two hours, or more if you're swimming/
sweating, etc.

6. Avoid SPF foundation as your only protection. It's nearly
impossible to apply enough to get effective protection without
looking like you're wearing a makeup mask.

WHAT WE USE

Hair

Lisa: Aveda Sun Care
Protective Hair Veil.
Sophie: Philip Kingsley Sun
Shield.

Face

Lisa: Ultrasun Face Anti-
Ageing
SPF 50+ Tinted.
Sophie: Obagi Medical Sun
Shield Tint SPF 50.

Lips

Lisa: Ultrasun Lip Protection
SPF 30.
Sophie: Aesop Protective Lip
Balm SPF 30.

Non comedogenic SPF
(non-pore blocking)

Lisa: La Roche Posay Anthelios
XL Ultra Light Tinted Fluid
SPF 50.
Sophie: Glossier Daily
Sunscreen
SPF 30.

Post-SPF (aftersun)

Lisa: Aloe Pura Aloe Vera Gel.
Sophie: Vichy Idéal Soleil
Aftersun.

TRAVEL
TIPS

WE TRAVEL A LOT, FOR WORK AND PLEASURE,
SO WE'VE ACCRUED A LOT OF
TRAVEL HACKS THAT INCLUDE
BEAUTY AND BEYOND.
HERE'S OUR TOP TEN.

1. A great place to find the minis you didn't even know you needed are in subscription beauty boxes. Sometimes you get mini versions that aren't otherwise available. Genius.

2. Go to Duty Free at the airport and ask for some perfume testers. You'll have an entire fragrance wardrobe for your holiday without having to cart a single full-size bottle with you.

3. If you're flying long-haul and you get the socks and eye mask, keep them for your future travel kit. Or home use. Lisa can often be seen in red Virgin socks with her workout trainers.

4. Invest in a super-comforting travel tracksuit. This can be hoodie and leggings, or coordinating knit jogger and top, basically something that feels comfortable and you feel good in. Save it for holiday so you feel special when you put it on.

5. Pack a lightweight, crease-free outfit in your hand luggage in case it's roasting hot when you get off the plane. Lisa takes a playsuit (and a swimsuit), Sophie takes a jersey mini skirt.

6. Buy a tiny cheap stand for your phone or tablet. Game-changer for hands-free plane entertainment.

7. Check in as soon as you can to get seats between the wings and the front. Less turbulence and you get off quicker!

8. If you're scared of flying (like Sophie), try listening to your favourite song with noise-cancelling headphones for take off. It masks the scary changing engine noises and by the time it's finished you'll be straightened out and in the air.

9. This Works Deep Sleep Pillow Spray is amazing. Spray it when you get to your seat. Your fellow passengers will also appreciate the calming effects!

10. If you're going long-haul, take your pillow from home. Yes, it's an extra thing to carry, but oh my goodness it makes the journey about 100% nicer, plus you can use it on your hotel bed, too.

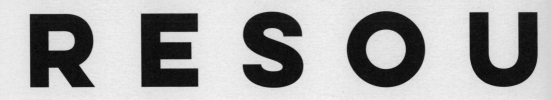

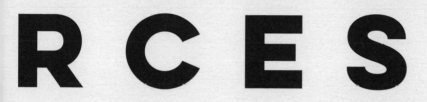

WHERE TO SHOP

SEPHORA
The OG beauty mecca for exclusives, trend edits and amazing own brand, too.

BOOTS
A British national health and beauty treasure with the best loyalty programme in the land.

SUPERDRUG
Best for affordable and entry-level beauty.

SPACE NK
Best for a bespoke curation of luxury makeup, hair- and skincare.

LOOK FANTASTIC
Comprehensive stock and amazing deals.

CULT BEAUTY
Famous for their cult finds, obviously.

FEEL UNIQUE
Easy access to the latest new and trending beauty products.

BEAUTY BAY
Great for finding Instagram-friendly products and brands.

NET A PORTER
The ultimate luxury edit and international exclusives.

BIRCHBOX
The subscription service we go to for the best minis.

SELFRIDGES
A slick beauty bonanza with all the top brands you can think of.

LIBERTY
For insiders, with the most coveted, niche and luxury buys.

HARVEY NICHOLS
The place for brand exclusives and international high-end finds.

WHAT
TO BUY

THESE ARE THE PRODUCTS WE SHOUT-OUT
IN THESE PAGES – YOU DON'T NEED
THEM ALL, BUT TRY OUT WHAT YOU
LIKE THE SOUND OF.

SKIN

Aloe Pura Aloe Vera Gel
Avene Skin Recovery Cream
Brazilian Bum Bum Cream
Cetaphil Cleanser
Downy Wrinkle Releaser
Egyptian Magic All Purpose Cream
Elemis Hydra-Boost Serum
Elemis Pro-Collagen Cleansing Balm
Glossier Daily Sunscreen SPF 30
Hada Labo Tokyo Skin Plumping Gel Cream
La Roche Posay Effaclar IA
La Roche Posay Thermal Spring Water Face Mist
MAC Prep + Prime Fix +
Mario Badescu Facial Spray with Aloe Herbs and Rosewater
Milk Makeup Cooling Water
Neal's Yard Remedies White Tea Facial Mist
Obagi Medical Sun Shield Tint SPF 50
Sudocrem
SkinCeuticals Hydrating B5 and CE Ferulic
The Body Shop Seaweed Oil-Control Gel Cream
The Ordinary 100% Organic Cold-Pressed Rosehip Seed Oil
TIME BOMB Cosmetics Holiday In a Bottle
Trilogy Rosehip Oil Light Blend
Ultrasun Face Anti-Ageing SPF 50+ Tinted
Ultrasun Sports Spray
Urban Decay All Nighter
XL Ultra Light Tinted Fluid SPF 50
Vichy Idéal Soleil Aftersun

BASE

bareMinerals Invisible Light Translucent Powder Duo
bareMinerals Original Foundation SPF 15
bareMinerals Pure Transformation Night Treatment
BECCA Backlight Priming Filter
Benefit Hello Happy Soft Blur Foundation
Benefit High Beam
Charlotte Tilbury Beach Stick in Las Salinas
Charlotte Tilbury Magic Away Liquid Concealer
Hourglass Ambient Light
La Roche Posay Anthelios XL Ultra Light Tinted Fluid
NARS Radiant Creamy Concealer
Paula's Choice Shine Stopper

BROWS

Benefit 24 Hour Brow Setter
Benefit Brow Contour Pro
Benefit Gimme Brow+

EYES

Benefit BADgal BANG!
Benefit Roller Lash
Charlotte Tilbury Luxury Palette The Golden Goddess
Clarins 4-colour Pen for Eyes and Lips
Clinique Lash Power Mascara
Dior Diorshow On Stage Liner
EcoStardust Biodegradable Glitter
Glossier Lash Slick
Hourglass Scattered Light Glitter Eyeshadow
Karla Cosmetics Glitter
Laura Mercier Caviar Stick Eye Colour in Taupe
MAC Chromagraphic Pencil in Genuine Orange
NYX Professional Makeup Wonder Pencil
Paintglow Glitter Gel
Pat McGrath Mothership II Sublime Palette
Pixi Beauty LashLift 188
Stila Magnificent Metals Glitter & Glow Liquid Eye Shadow in
    Rose Gold Retro
The Gypsy Shrine
Urban Decay 24/7 Glide-On Eye Pencil
YSL Mascara in Blue

LIPS

Aesop Protective Lip Balm SPF 30
Aquaphor Lip Repair
Benefit Benetint
Bobbi Brown Creamy Matte Lip Color in Red Carpet
Christian Dior Rouge Dior Lip Colour in 999
Crayola Lip Crayon in Red and Bronze
Dior Addict Lip Glow
Fresh Sugar Sport Treatment
Gatineau Perfection Ultime Nourishing Lip Balm
Laura Mercier Velour Exteme Matte Lip in Stylin
MAC Lady Danger
MAC Ruby Woo
Maybelline Color Sensational Matte in Craving Coral
Pat McGrath Mattetrance Lipstick in Elson
Rouge Allure Velvet in First Light by Chanel

Rouge Velvet The Lipstick in Rubi's Cute by Bourjois
Ultrasun Lip Protection SPF 30
Ultrasun Lip Protection SPF 30
Winky Lux Jelly pH Lip Balm
YSL Rouge Pur Couture in Le Orange

HAIR

Aveda Sun Care Protective Hair Veil
Bumble & Bumble Brilliantine
Colab Dry Shampoo
L'Oreal Elnett Hairspray
Larry King A Social Life For Your Hair
Living Proof Perfect Hair Day Dry Shampoo
OGX Nourishing Coconut Milk Anti-Breakage Serum
Onira Organics The Onira Oil
Percy & Reed The Perfect Blow Dry Makeover Spray
Philip Kingsley Sun Shield
Redken Wind Blown 05 Finishing Spray
Sam McKnight Cool Girl Barely There Texture Mist

TOOLS AND ACCESSORIES

ASOS Oversized Velvet Bow
bareMinerals Original Powder Foundation Brush
Beautyblender
Benefit Angled Brow Brush and Spoolie
Charlotte Tilbury Powder & Sculpt Brush
Crown Eye Brush C163
DAFNI Hair Straightening Brush
GHD Curve Classic Wave Wand
Lee Stafford's Chopstick Styler
Louise Constad Lip Brush
MAC 316 Lip Brush
Real Techniques PowderBleu Soft Shadow Brush
Syd Pin by Syd Hayes
Tangle Teezer
Wayne Goss Brush 10 Cheek Brush
Zoeva Concealer Brush

TREATMENTS

Cowshed Udderly Gorgeous Body
Elemis Peaceful Pregnancy Massage
This Works Deep Sleep Pillow Spray

THANK YOU

S.B. Hi Mum and Dad. I would like to thank you first, partly because I'm always thankful for you both and I always always will be, and partly because I know you will love seeing your own 'thank you' in my own book.

Thank you also to my husband, Mr. B, who had to put up with many shouty Instagram Live backchats and regular kazoo playing when he was trying to work in the kitchen. I love you.

Thank you to Stephanie Milner, Laura Russell, Adam Hale and Pete Pedonomou for bringing our vision to life in these pages.

L.P.D. And for putting up with our crazy schedules. Thank you so much! And to Sue for the writing retreat in the rain.

But mostly... Thank you to Prosecco and coffee. OK, just kidding...

Mostly, thank you to my cats, Woody, Columbo and Coco. OK, still kidding; mostly, thank you to my main woman, my beauty partner in crime, my co-conspirator and now co-author(!), my beautiful and talented friend Lisa Potter-Dixon. So this was fun, huh?

To our OG Insta fam.

Yes! The actual inspiration. How could I forget!

Thank you for tuning into #BCB and for loving it so much. Without you lot, this book wouldn't have been possible.

Soph, I have to say, there is no one else I would have wanted to write this beauty of a book with. Thank you for being the best friend, co-writer and camembert maker. Even if you don't know the right order of the rainbow(!). We've done it, girl.
I'm so proud of us.

Theo, I mean, without you, nothing would be possible. LYF.

Snoop, Diddy and Kimmy, You da best.

My friends and family, you know who you are. Thank you for always supporting my crazy ideas.

Do we get to go on holiday now Soph?! #backpackbeauty?!

INDEX